# CODE-ONE DANCING

# CODE-ONE DANCING

MEDICINE

MURDER

REVENGE

FICTION
BY

MICHAEL ELLMAN

# CODE-ONE
## DANCING





Portions of *Code-One Dancing* have been published in different forms in *Front Porch Review*, *Third Wednesday*, the *Hektoen International Journal* and *Black Heart* magazine. The author wishes to thank the editors of those journals.

Windy City Publishers
2118 Plum Grove Road #349
Rolling Meadows, IL 60008
www.windycitypublishers.com

Published in the United States of America

Library of Congress Control Number:
2016953439

ISBN:
978-1-941478-33-2

WINDY CITY PUBLISHERS

Chicago

*This book is dedicated to my family:*
*Roberta, Bruce, Carol, Brett, Fred, Benjamin, Charles, John, and Lydia.*

# PART ONE

# ONE

## *Fall 1960*

Blue-collar residential, the area should have been safe: no FOR SALE signs, Old World family names plastered on store windows, and crabgrass sprayed, speared, and pulled daily. Front lawns were flat, as if elves had descended in the pre-dawn and taken a level to them. Police in the neighborhood headed home, not searching for bad guys loitering in the shadows.

The intersection was quiet, the corner diner only open for breakfast and lunch, and dark except for the neon sign rhythmically flashing GOOD FOOD. The dry cleaner next door that starched and ironed my shirts, washed my slacks, and offered S&H Green Stamps remained shuttered for the evening. Red brick apartment buildings stretched down the street as if forever, the murky evening-glow merging them into one. A quick drive around the block and I could find a parking space, a welcome relief after a long day and evening at the hospital.

Sleep would arrive quickly, exhaustion a potent sedative, but still there was time for a paragraph or two of *Cecil's Medicine* and perhaps a moment for a few pages of Dickens. No need for victuals, the hospital cafeteria food was gratis for residents after 7 p.m. Perhaps, in my future life, I would supply the hospital with their barrels of macaroni and cheese and gain wealth.

He caught my attention because he was big and smiling and close and speaking to my face, saying "Hey, Doc," followed by a fist straight into my gut. I didn't fall backward as my body bent in two, because the little guy, almost invisible in the dusk, the one wielding the big slab of lumber, propped me up from behind. Then a major-league wallop to my mid-back. Lou Gehrig and the Babe would have approved—the hit located in this guy's demented idea of a strike zone, accompanied by another punch from Mr. Big. I crumpled to the ground, sickness in my stomach, bile working its way up, pain extending down to my suddenly and inconveniently paralyzed legs.

The little fellow with the baseball cap and White Sox jacket raised his bat to shoulder level rhythmically working his fingers on the handle á-la Ernie Banks. "Doc, whaddya want, anklesorknees?" His words were mixed with spittle and in an accent I didn't decipher until months later.

"Anklesorknees, huh?"

"The fuck you're saying?" I mumbled, adding a feeble, "Asshole," accompanied by my vomit. Lessons in toughness learned from my father—a big mistake. And there was no point in telling Mr. Baseball that Ernie played for the Cubs.

The bat descended at light speed on my left patella, too late for me to ask for "ankle please," now that his muttering made sense. The crunch of the fracture was audible, but no sound came from me, as a boot from my original friend cracked my ribs. Always the doctor, I prayed for no lung puncture from the misplaced bones, as my back settled down onto the craggy sidewalk.

God in his mercy limits the amount of pain you feel just before passing out, and from a great distance away, perhaps even from the surface of the rising moon edging its way over the skyscrapers clustered in the east, the little guy, floating in space, with spittle but no acrimony, mouthed: "*That's for Betty.*"

# TWO

I awoke lying in a general surgery bed in my own hospital. Familiar white walls bordering the old-time sash windows sealed shut by layers of paint told me I was safe. The morning sun filtered through the tattered window blinds, yellowed by age and resting at an acute angle, provided streaks of light on my supine body. One of my arms was dark and the other sparkled. Skilled fingers adjusted the intravenous bottle hopefully supplemented with morphine. Pain from the chest tube—the damn rib fracture did tear the lung after all—vied with the pain from my kneecap.

"More morphine," I said. My first words in what seemed like a week.

"Awake, are we, Doctor?"

My good fortune, I had a nurse with an advanced degree.

"You're lucky some neighbors came by and interrupted the beating," she continued. "They didn't even take your wallet. You're really fortunate. My sister was robbed of her purse and engagement ring. They nearly took her finger off, mind you, and after they got everything they wanted, they hit her in the nose. Five stitches, no less. They didn't even touch your handsome face. Dr. Ted, you were double lucky."

"Condolences to your sister," I breathlessly said to the motor mouthed Clara Barton, "but please limit the chitchat and get the morphine."

Maybe my words annoyed Nurse, because she straightened the bedcovers, shaking my knee to and fro, just to remind me that the bone was shattered. Then she started on my face, finishing the morning cleanup, as all good nurses must, using a raggedy, soap-encrusted washcloth left over from the Civil War, Clara's initials likely sewn on the back. The suds burning my eyes were therapeutic because my shouts expanded my lung.

My face was pristine when I awakened again. Darkness had taken over. It was night, but which night? My wristband read *Tadeusz Shluzkinski, M.D., third year medical resident*, and that was me, as best I could remember. No matter the day, because there, inches from my eyes, was Sophie. I was triple lucky.

Floating in this drug-induced fugue state, it was the sixth dimension, the one after euphoria, otherwise it would be the Fox and the Gingerbread Boy routine that Sophie had heard too often. "*Come closer*," I'd say, "*I can't hear what you're saying*," and I'd pull her down until our lips met.

"Ted, I was so worried about you. I'm so thankful you're all right," she said, accompanied by a Sophie smile. My heart was gladdened by her proximity. "You're my Gregory Peck," she said. Tears clouded her eyes. "Mount Kilimanjaro sits right there behind the curtain, majestic and snow capped, and me, Sophie, not Susan Hayward, will nurse you back to health."

Sophie adjusted my new glasses, thin brown frames, bookish-looking. Her hands lingered. She wanted me to see her eyes, she said. Her fingers moved to my wrist, a nurse thing, feeling for my pulse—there was no need to, a monitor above my head ticked away the beats—but her touch told me how good it was to be alive. And what was all that about Gregory Peck? He died with gangrene, for chrissakes, reliving his failures, while roasting in the tropical sun. Sure it was Susan Hayward fluttering around him, but as for me, I'd go out banging Ava Gardner.

Howard visited. We hugged and shared smiles, our minds meshed finer than tines in a Swiss timepiece. Having shared medical school and residency training, we could have been twins. We were medicine's Two Step Brothers with Four Feet of Rhythm singing and dancing together in our off hours, kind of like tap dancing—it attracted girls.

"I should have been there the night of the beating. The two of us can take anybody," Howard whispered. His chest seemed to swell as he spoke. He needed the catharsis.

Doctors don't get assaulted. My injuries had been flashed across the local papers. Sergeant Esposito insisted on an interrupted drug deal. His murder investigation of Betty's death wasn't going anywhere, and premature publicity wouldn't help.

The photograph of me, meticulously excised from my official class picture, with bored demeanor and borrowed tie pulled upward too tight, wrinkling the cords under my chin, reassured Mother. "*Likely to fully recover*," the caption read. Tell that to my pain centers. The neighborhood watch committee had already formed and I would be the honorary chairman.

The sergeant didn't think more violence was likely, but he'd assign a squad car team to keep an eye on me.

"Not as if that helps a lot," he intoned. "Last year we had this goof under protective custody. He demanded the works: twenty-four-hour protection, a different apartment, a fake mustache, a new hairpiece—Lord, what a cheesy looking item that was—and he wanted a bulletproof vest.

"They dragged him out of the washroom window at his favorite steak house and dumped him in the lake, while my guys watched the game on the upstairs television, the one over the bar, just one beer apiece I'd told them. Billy Pierce versus Whitey Ford, eighth inning, three to nothing, good guys winning, can you believe it?

"Ever try swimming wearing a fifteen-pound protective vest? We found the guy lying twenty-five feet below his toupee. The thingamajig was like a harbor buoy, bobbing up and down in the water. Like an apple in a tub for dunking. You know, like the game the kids play at birthday parties." The sergeant bellowed a hearty laugh.

"Doc, here's my thinking," he said. "You got payback for insisting on the autopsy on Betty Schmidt against the family's wishes, and then you coming to see me claiming she was murdered by her husband. Tim Schmidt's high up in the crime world and you don't cross those guys." The sergeant's index finger tapped in time with his spoken words on the bed rail. "When his goons are serious, they don't offer you options and they leave their bat at home to free up their shooting hand. You were lucky."

If I could have taken all those "luckys" to the bank, I'd be some rich doctor.

# THREE

Mrs. B handed me a gift card. "Open it, Doctor, it's from me and my cafeteria workers," she said, working on a rarely offered smile. The card pictured a yellow Labrador with a kerchief around its neck, drool spiraling downward from its open mouth—the kind of greeting card you see in notion shops all around the world. I didn't understand the significance of the hound. "*Dog*" had never appeared on the hospital menu. Inside the card, the prize, a handwritten "*get well doctor*," spelled correctly in a third grade scrawl with a leaky ballpoint pen, the blotchy words slanted in several directions, and attached was a hospital cafeteria gift certificate good for three regular-sized coffees.

Mrs. B couldn't explain the significance of the offer of three, except any fool knew three was better than one or two. "Just regular-sized coffee, not jumbo, no toast or sweet rolls, and don't take too many sugar packets and napkins. And if you have any on-call coupons you won't need while you're laid up, we'll take them."

"Thanks, Mrs. B," I said.

Mrs. Gail, the dumpy, precisely dressed *de facto* ruler of the Department of Medicine, arrived next. I rarely saw her outside the chief's office. She offered condolences regarding the "accident" and the familiar mantra of how lucky I was.

"You're so efficient," I told her. "Every day I'm not comatose, I thank the stars and moon for your devotion to the hospital and the medical residents, and especially for the attention you provide me."

Shedding my obsequiousness as if it were the dog's saliva from the gift card, she outlined her plans for me—one week recuperating at home, then a two-week rotation reading X-rays where I would sit quietly with the radiology wizards, regaining my strength before returning to my hematology month.

"And," she said, the word was underscored as a smile appeared on her stern face, "the Department of Medicine, pending hospital approval of course, will arrange transportation for you back and forth from your home until you're able to drive, what with your leg in a splint and all." She tapped my knee with her index finger—t he pressure sending shock waves up my thigh.

Mother and stepfather Harry flew in from Florida to sit with their sonny boy. My face was showered with kisses, combined with multi-ethnic blessings. Then came the weepy stuff. Their concerns tempered by the happiness of seeing me move and talk and laugh even. Gold necklaces danced over my nose, intersecting one another like Japanese box kites crowding a holiday afternoon sky. Mother standing on the left, Harry on the right, leaning over me, they were handsome people, her delicate gold cross intertwining with his Star of David.

❖ ❖ ❖

My father, the butcher, was the brilliant one, an autodidact, polymath, Polish tradesman, descendent of Nicolaus Copernicus, Marie Sklodowska-Curie and Fryderyk Chopin. He explained the math, corrected my grammar and checked my English. Killed when I was fourteen—a hold-up at a gas station when the kids ran out and demanded his keys. He wouldn't have given them up for anything in the world. I like to think my father knew how much I loved him, but then, you never know that for sure—doubts that linger even now at awkward intervals.

Mother married Harry one year later—the friendly pharmacist who owned the neighborhood drugstore with the white marble-topped soda fountain serving chocolate sodas with crushed walnuts dotting the whipped cream. Mother was a pigeon for chocolate sodas topped with walnuts and whipped cream, and *voilà*, Harry was over for dinner, then a picnic, then a movie, then the Las Vegas nuptials.

Older than Mother, a happy professional, Harry came with no complaints about life, pleased with this his first marriage and his wise choice. He introduced me to the *New York Times*, the *New Yorker*, and *The Atlantic*, a literary universe

I adopted with greedy pleasure. Harry was medium height with a tendency to being heavy; he was sports-minded, but not an athlete. Still he admired the gap-toothed smile and fearsome slap shot of Bobby Hull, the Golden Jet, and we greeted each other with wrists cocked and the cry—"it's a goal."

We moved north and I started an academic high school, leaving my friends and a neighborhood wrestling with trouble. Average size for my age entering puberty, but as if by magic, I filled out and grew big, developed muscles, had arms, rolled up my sleeves, made cuffs to hold a cigarette pack, although of course I wasn't allowed to smoke.

With a Polish name and a Jewish stepfather, I stood out like a visitor from Neptune, or more likely Monaco or Lichtenstein, countries discovered in the stamp albums these kids pored over. My prowess in sports and ability to comb my hair straight brought acceptance; Tadeusz Shluzkinski became Ted S.

❖ ❖ ❖

Dr. Rhimes came by to say hello. He was our chief. His noble countenance parted the Red Sea of visitors and his chair was emptied of detritus by my Clara Barton, who shooed everyone away. He talked about my future while shaking his head with condolences about my beating.

"You solve problems well, you're intuitive, and when you focus your thoughts, you achieve good things," he said, but there was no mention of rewarding me with the Department of Medicine's Annual Prize or even an offer of future employment. Perhaps it was an oversight.

"Talk to me soon. Consider further training. Get well," he declared. A handshake, a pat on my shoulder, nothing on my knee, relieved to have completed this visit. Now it was off to his pipe, Scotch, and mellower chores.

During the twilight between my morphine and pain, I did think about my future. I would discuss it with him. The chief didn't realize how much he was worshipped.

❖ ❖ ❖

Our medical school conferences were euphemistically entitled "Grand Rounds," and today for a change, it lived up to the name. Dr. Rhimes, the chief of medicine, was good, even enthusiastic, his talk understandable at our primitive level of expertise. He laced his discourse with words like *motif* and *repertoire* and *reductionistic*; it was similar to reading a Gore Vidal essay—a dictionary splayed open on our laps was a necessity.

Doctors talked about their "cutting edge" research, the epitome of their achievements. But most of the time their successes reminded us more of the science behind the huge slicing machine at the noisy delicatessen counter, carving thin slices of pastrami from a fatty amorphous concretion, slice by slice, precise and reproducible perhaps, but not innovative.

The chief presented new ideas about thyroid hormone and how different constitutive messengers interacted with receptors on non-thyroid tissue. A difficult concept for me to comprehend, but I liked the word *constitutive* and underlined it in my notes.

I waited around after the lecture and asked the chief if he would schedule an interview for me. I was beginning to apply for medical residencies and he directed one of the best. Smart people who were good teachers were rare, and I pictured the two of us bonding over our shared brilliance, mentor and student, me and the chief.

We met later that week after I spent several painful hours researching his genius. I talked his talk, smiling, fawning, back straight, eyes straightforward and intersecting his, shirt buttons lined up correctly, just as they had taught me in interview class. I was accepted at his institution for my three-year internal medicine residency. It proved to be the pinnacle of our relationship.

❖ ❖ ❖

The troubles began in my first week of residency training. I was assigned to the emergency room, a cluster of small, dark rooms, too cramped for the clientele the hospital served, but similar to all the money losing endeavors at this institution not likely to be fixed soon. Like most service industries, hospitals were a mixture of the old and new. Psychiatry was new, surgery with the money-generating suites was new, but the ER was old, Roosevelt vintage old—Theodore Roosevelt old.

July 4th and we're mobbed with patients. I was a seasoned medical resident after only three days down there. The stink of the place, the wounds, the antiseptics, the unwashed, were already muffled by familiarity.

The outside air was fat with smog and heat, the motionless sky the color of pale white wine plus splotches of ragged-edged clouds that offered no shade and resembled fragments of a difficult, too-many-piece picture puzzle. In addition to the knife wounds and hypochondriacs crowding every corner, we entertained a coterie of asthmatics, each one more short of breath than the next, their holiday hopes dashed by the heavy, unhealthy air of the early Midwestern heat wave.

Only if you were young and fair with a superficial nothing on the upper inner thigh or anywhere on the breast tissue, guaranteed to be non-infectious by the triage nurse, could you expect prompt and enthusiastic attention. Otherwise it was close your eyes, moan, stretch out, and wait.

A middle-aged guy, too big, legs jutting over the table, and intruding into the aisle lay still in the priority examining room. He differed from the other denizens that crowded the ER because of the ice-pick handle that stuck out from his left ear, the long metallic business end snug tight, deep in his brain. How did such a big person come out second-best in an altercation? We were waiting for him to die when his family barged in.

"You're not going to do anything for him, just let him lie there?" His missus wailed in my face, squeezing past the security guard who was too busy restraining the remainder of the clan. "How old are you, anyway?" she asked, her eyes abutting mine, picking up the lack of wrinkles and fault lines, astutely reading my inexperience in treating ice-pick trauma to the deep brain. "Get someone in here who knows what to do," she screamed, pointing an accusatory finger my way, while my hands nervously stroked the stethoscope hanging from my neck.

I paged the neurosurgery resident on call.

"You want me to do what?" he yelled, his words as hard as the frozen outer planets. "If I come down there, I'm going to pull out that ice pick and insert it up your nose, you nitwit. He's going to die!" His tirade followed by a long pause until he decided to be helpful: "Send him to X-ray!" he commanded.

"To X-ray! Send him to X-ray—is that what you said?" I shouted back into the phone—my turn for disbelief.

X-rays would only confirm what we already knew. This poor schnook had an ice-pick lodged in his brain. Just then, as if sensing our animus, Mr. Ice-pick in his Brain, awakened to say hello, ask for a sip of water—he was thirsty he said, very polite like, before returning to his coma.

"Why in God's name should I send the patient to X-ray?" I asked the neurosurgeon, not at all startled by the patient's momentary lucidity. "It won't accomplish a thing."

"By the time he's dumped on a cart, hustled down the halls and tunnel to Radiology, dragged off and rolled onto the X-ray table for a skull film series, and then positioned this way and that, he'll be dead, and it will be the radiologist's problem." And he hung up.

The nurse handed me the completed X-ray requisition, requiring only my signature. I should solicit her opinion more often. The missus and family marched out, the security guard gave me a thumbs-up and that was that. Radiology took the X-rays as ordered and the ice-pick guy died.

I've kept the radiology report, now yellowing with age, but ever-so fresh in my memory: *There's motion artifact, but it appears that an ice-pick lies completely within brain tissue, involving mainly the brain stem, temporal cortex and penetrating through the third ventricle into the opposite hemisphere. <u>Please note this constitutes a medical emergency</u>.*

The ambulance pulled up, lights flashing, the wail of the siren lingering over the hum of the busy ER. A pimply-faced medic rushed in and grabbed my arm just as I was starting an intravenous drip of aminophylline into one of the wheezing teenagers and told me to come with him "stat." He pulled my arm with an ungloved hand, no attention to sterility, just in a hurry, and the hell with my dyspneic adolescents.

The medic wanted me to sign the death certificate on a decomposed body that had spent weeks floating in the lake and had just washed up onto the crowded beach, terrifying holiday revelers and captivating their sand castle building youngsters who were already bored with the day's activities. The children were now able to expand their show-and-tell repertoire while the spectacle played out in the morning heat.

"Sign here, Doc." The medic dismissively handed me his pen, while I viewed the bloated remains. "And we're off to the County Morgue and then lunch, so please hustle."

I grabbed the medic, high up on the chest, my hands and his shirt tight on his neck, shutting off his breathing. His thick glasses with the white surgical tape patching the plastic frames slipped precariously to the tip of his nose a few degrees off-center, as I lifted him onto the side of the ambulance.

"Asshole, if you ever drag me out again to see someone who's dead longer than a day"—my mouth inches from his face, but not too close to his acne—"I'm going to rearrange your face and that would be an improvement." I dropped him to the ground, leaving a life-sized, dust-angel silhouette on the passenger-side panel.

I signed the form and went back to care for the living.

Who would have thought this minor disagreement would be reported to the city commissioner of health and the hospital president with copies of the complaint to my cherished chief of medicine? Two and a half years later, the lawsuit was still pending, while the slob collected disability pay.

On top of that nonsense, the neurosurgery resident suggested that I receive further training in managing head trauma. Meticulously spelled out, the official letter was typed on Department of Neurosurgery stationery lined on the left margin with the names of their luminaries, co-signed by their chief, and hand-carried to the Department of Medicine and Mrs. Gail.

# FOUR

"Do you want to get laid?"

I was in a drug-induced sleep, deeper than the subway as it traveled south under the river bisecting our downtown, slowly recovering from the Mr. Big and Mr. Baseball slugging party. The morphine sluiced into my median-cubital vein at a steady rate.

Howard was talking to me. I couldn't awaken, but that wasn't so bad. Who doesn't want to get laid."

❖ ❖ ❖

My best buddy ever, Howard was too often quiet and sometimes underestimated, but hidden beneath the placid demeanor lay the charm and wit of a courtier. The scion of a wealthy East Coast family, his Ivy League school attendance and his piano virtuosity made him an unlikely Midwestern state school student. And he was smart. He could attend any school in the country except for several endearing details.

Soft drug use was recorded in the police blotter several times, minor misdemeanors for sure, but his financial good fortune allowed the largesse of distributing pot to his less-fortunate buddies. When his automobile packed with the starting five from the basketball team, juniors and seniors, all semi-stoned, crashed into the town square, well, you can picture the uproar.

Up until then, the Paul Revere monument had been pristine except for the chin rubbing, wearing the metal down to its shiny core, considered good luck in that part of the world. The car's impact removed the patriot's right leg from the knee down. It's known as a "BK amputation" or "BKA" in medical parlance, while at the same time the automobile, now of police interest, ran over the sheriff's boxer dog that in all rights shouldn't have been outside without a leash, nor should have been urinating on Paul's foot for that matter, and certainly not so late in the night. They're short lived anyway, boxer dogs, and squat and homely, but apparently in this instance, beloved, because Howard spent a night and a day in the village jail and even the two-hundred-dollar-an-hour lawyer couldn't abort the pending conviction.

Howard never expressed pride in his youthful misdeeds, or remorse either for that matter. He learned from his mistakes, never distributing marijuana again to basketball acquaintances, only to loved ones, and I was included.

❖ ❖ ❖

It was the Sunday before we started our residency training. We were revved up like college students on an amphetamine high before the final examinations. Introductions and tours were finished. The next day I would start in the emergency room and Howard in the intensive care unit. Today, we were taking in the sights and sounds of our great city.

I stared at a Rothko in the bustling Art Institute, and smiled at the shapely young lady standing nearby, with blonde hair the color of late-summer sweet corn and form-fitting, soft blue jeans. Isolated from the turmoil of the packed gallery, we were concentrating on the magical rectangles and the astonishing colors.

"Excuse me, miss," I said, my fingers pointing to the Rothko. "What message is the artist sending you? I always want to know what beautiful people think."

She turned to me, her glance thoroughly sizing me up. My pulse quickened.

"What message?" she repeated, moving closer. She was tall, nearly my height, and I sensed her warmth. "You tell me," she said.

I paused for a moment, my left hand stroking my chin in faux concentration, before replying to my own query.

"He's channeling me creative love, beauty and *gemütlichkeit*. By the way," I asked, "is there any place where we can get some good coffee, ponder the great lessons of life, and hold hands?"

The trouble with the drug-induced dreams is their end. Their middle is also scary.

From her generous mouth, she told me that before we went anywhere we needed to settle on a price.

"It's one hundred dollars if we go to my room. If that doesn't work, how about playing a little baseball," as she slowly extracted a full-sized Louisville Slugger cleverly hidden inside her diminutive purse.

I yelled for Howard, but my cries fell on deaf ears.

The red and orange rectangles of the Rothko faded as my sleep lightened. I was sitting in the graveyard at Grover's Corners discussing my future with Nurse Sophie and Mr. Baseball, my Iowa beauty drifting away, not interested in a deadbeat with dangling chest tubes.

My dream was further interrupted by the sound of the afternoon snack cart. The squeal of the never-oiled wheels and the *ding* and then the *jingle-jangle* of the old-fashioned bicycle handlebar bell announced its arrival. Volunteer ladies wearing their green-colored smocks over formal attire, aggressively offered tiny morsels of sweets and liquids, but were careful not to get too close to the inmates.

"May I have a muffin and a soda?" I asked. My appetite was beginning to return.

But for some reason the ladies only offered counsel.

"Shape-up, you ninny, get better, get even, get tough!" It was a chorus from the Valkyries.

And they were correct.

I thought about my patient, Betty Schmidt, and I thought about revenge for her murder, and payback for my beating.

# PART TWO

# ONE

## *Summer 1960*

"I know what time it is, Mrs. B, but I'm still on-call." I was trying to pay for my coffee with the on-call vouchers and Mrs. B, who had hassled me for almost two years now, told me it was morning and I couldn't use them. "My beeper is still on admitting mode, want to see it?" I told her, but I didn't bother tugging it out of my pocket.

"It's too late," she said. There was no acrimony yet.

"I spent my entire night in this hellhole of a hospital, working my body to the bare-bone trying to do good and I need coffee." It was my usual counter to her negativity, but today was different; the despair was real.

There's no one around for a doctor to talk to when bad things happen during the night. You can't pick-up the phone at 2 a.m. and ask Sophie or Howard or the chief: "Where did I screw up? Why did the patient die? Should I have given more medication, or less, or none at all?" You're on your own and when your decisions crash, they weigh heavily. And I was taking it out on Mrs. B.

Who cares what her real name was, as she stiffed us for our change, sitting like a queen at the register, growing a bigger ass—while compulsively counting every penny and coupon as if they were her precious tarot cards of doom meant for her many enemies. Queen Liliuokalani resurrected and deposited in the hospital cafeteria, her last opportunity to resurrect a monarchy. And it was happening here in the basement of my hospital and she was yelling at me, while preparing for her monthly luau with leftover food crammed inside carved pineapple rinds.

I knew somewhere there was a soft spot in her shifty mind and I knew her routines by rote.

"Do you want me to call the manager?" she asked, chin working up and down. If her stool was any higher, she would be loftier than the lifeguards at the North Avenue Beach, scanning her domain and bellowing orders through a bullhorn to the miscreants below.

I said the "*go jump in the lake*" to myself and flashed Mrs. B my winning smile, still capable of fabricating it, although it wasn't even 7 a.m.

"Well, I'm the manager and the on-call coupons are no good in the morning, Mr. Big Shot Doctor, and my name isn't Mrs. B," and she laughed and let me go.

"Next time, order chamomile tea with lemon," she yelled at my back, as I departed her domain. "It'll be good for your wiseass attitude," giving me her standard parting salvo, while I pantomimed the words along with her. Ordinarily, I'd be pleased with my arrogance, but not today.

Funny, when Mrs. B, the *B* for *Bitch* of course, my contribution, wasn't there, I missed her. Sick a whole week once, cough and flu, you'd think working at a hospital, people wouldn't cough on you, but she was a bulls-eye for phlegm, sitting there at the register, leaning in your face, her rancor bringing her close—and she lived for rancor. I phoned her at home and offered to bring coffee and hot buttered lemonade with honey. She laughed and told me not to worry. "There's plenty of chamomile tea in my cupboard, and don't palm off any on-call coupons in my absence." croaking the words before disconnecting. I tried, but even her less-gifted associates wouldn't accept them.

The cafeteria, probably not much different from any other hospital cafeteria, had transformed like magic into our warming house, our sustenance provider, our refuge; the familiarity of the metal chair legs scraping across the pitted linoleum floor, the Don Ho folk-songs, the steamed everything, the close air, the shrill noise, it was our sanctuary placed just below the six stories of bedlam above it. The well-heeled, the streetwalkers, the down on their luck, all the hungry people participated in this little democracy, because Mrs. B yelled at all of them. Lysol-clean, but messy, nothing permanent, paper plates, napkins thinner than toilet paper, plastic everything else, but the memories were indelible.

I didn't ask Mrs. B how they made the coffee so thick and black and devoid of taste. No taste at all, yet as dark as Midnight the Cat. The coffee aroma combined with the piquant smell drifting over from the pyramid of bacon slices, only ten cents apiece, each strip, perfectly crisp and uniform, an epicurean necessity for hungry doctors after an exhausting and unhappy evening on call.

The bacon drew a big crowd when the shift changed, satisfying caloric and fat demands. But, if you wanted to eat healthy or you liked cinnamon sprinkles in your coffee, the hospital cafeteria was not your place.

# TWO

I left a message for Mrs. Gail telling her I needed to see the chief. I would be at their office at 7:30. They'd both be sipping their own brewed coffee, by reputation delicious, but I would never discover that firsthand. Our adversarial relationship wouldn't improve after the morning visit.

"Good morning, Mrs. Gail, is the chief in?"

Her light red lipstick in place and wearing a clean, crisp long-sleeved white blouse buttoned to the neck; a short skirt, a perennial poor choice, revealing vein-mottled hefty legs, made more striking by a rim of blubber overhanging her knees. Yet, she was Gucci-shoed and proudly regal.

Mrs. Gail exhibited disdain without speaking. Darting eyes searched faces for weakness, before it was head down and back to her chores. She was working on a crossword puzzle or her horoscope or both I was sure, rather than a vital document for the board of directors or the chief, but she guarded her work well, and vigilantly protected her boss.

"Dr. Rhimes can't see you this morning, Dr. Ted," she told me with just a glimmer of a smirk, the three syllable "*Dr. Ted*" rolling out like a bad punch line and lasting longer than a Monday.

"The chief also can't see you this afternoon. Look at your next month's schedule and then discard it because he can't see you then either." There was no animosity, just facts, her head back down, her posture compact and assured, surveying her desk and the morning's chores.

"Mrs. Gail, it's a matter of life and death that I see the chief."

For my entire life I've wanted to say "*it's a matter of life or death*," and I said it, and it was actually true. It felt good.

Mrs. Gail had given me the worst schedule of any medical resident, so what further harm could she do to me for standing my ground?

"Ah, Doctor, could that be why Dr. Rosenthal and a Mr. Schmidt are calling the office every thirty seconds about an event that took place last night?" Her steely gray eyes fixed on me. "You must have been on call last night—right, Doctor? Maybe that explains all the turmoil this morning on what I thought was going to be a quiet and productive day. Now things are coming together." Her index finger pointed at me, eyes searching mine again, her words spilling out in staccato rhythm. "You were on call last night, weren't you? The phone hasn't stopped ringing, and now you want to provoke the chief. What kind of mischief have you created?"

"Mrs. Gail, has anyone told you how gorgeous you look when you're riled up? Does Mr. Gail know how lucky he is when he awakens every morning next to you, lips poised to caress your lovely mouth?" That hurt because it was public knowledge that Mr. Gail was screwing one of the nurses on the psychiatric unit.

My smile doesn't work on Mrs. Gail so I didn't bother with it as she stood up and high-heeled over to the chief's office. "He's here." Her thumb directed toward me.

"You can go in now Doctor, keep it brief, and thank you for the kind words about me and Mr. Gail."

My apologies were heartfelt, but silent.

❖ ❖ ❖

The antechamber with Mrs. Gail's desk and the chief's room were surprisingly small for the center of great power. The latter was made even smaller by the too-many bookcases lining the periphery and reaching the ceiling, crammed with well-thumbed journals and textbooks, orderly arranged by year of publication. The chief was orderly.

"Ted, sit down, while I get a notepad and pencil," spoken in a neutral and calm voice, while the chief prepared for this unscheduled interruption.

Medium height, fifty years old or so, his precise age a secret—heavy, but not soft, he was clean-shaven and academic-appearing with corduroy slacks, crisp with heavy starch. His brown laced shoes had worn plain tips shiny with polish, and soft rubber soles that allowed him to sneak up on his residents during unannounced strolls through the medical wards. The old-fashioned, bulky, black, thick-tubed stethoscope protruding from the left-hand side pocket of his herringbone jacket hanging from the spindly metal coat rack was the only symbol that the chief was a doctor as well as a scientist.

"Chief, I'm sorry to burst in like this and thanks in advance for your patience. Also, my thanks to Mrs. Gail for letting me see you on a moment's notice." Obsequiousness was never out of style when talking to the chief, plus, I was on solid ground. He needed to be kept up-to-date. And I needed to tap his wisdom.

His ties belied his academia—expensive, silk, stain-free, lightly lined, and knotted with the precision that mirrored his thinking. Favored residents reported that after several swigs of his single-malt Scotch, bottles of which rolled around in every desk drawer, lessons would be offered on necktie tying, demonstrating the intricacies of the Windsor and the four-in-hand.

Straight stem with a spacious bowl, his pipe was worn pale from years of handling. The sweet pungency of the aromatic tobacco, reminiscent of our feeble attempts to seduce freshman coeds at the Friday night smokers, promptly ignited with the downward flame of the lighter. The chief searched my face, his unwavering hazel eyes that could quickly shade dark and stern, fixed on mine. His eyebrows slanted upward, almost a startle response, followed by a nearly imperceptible sigh of contentment. The smoking ritual quieted unruly novices and allowed the chief time to formulate his wisdom and discern our strengths and weaknesses.

❖ ❖ ❖

"Betty Schmidt," I told the chief, "was a patient with lupus, hospitalized because of several days of abdominal pain that Dr. Rosenthal diagnosed as viral gastroenteritis, but getting no better with clear liquids and rest. Up until now, her lupus had been under control with modest doses of prednisone."

I gave the chief the medical information, even the minutiae, concisely and in order. Ever since the ninth-grade English class embarrassment, I carefully pictured my words before letting them fly. My speech center had become obfuscated by teenage hormones as I had substituted *ejaculate* for *calculate* during my out-loud recitation of Shakespeare.

"No one else was ill at home and these GI symptoms were new," I said. The chief nodded, taking notes, offering reassuring glances, gathering information by paying attention to my presentation, noting my inflections and word choices and simultaneously tapping in to his library of experience and wisdom.

"Her pulse was 100 and regular, temperature 101 degrees Fahrenheit and blood pressure 110/70. There were no rashes." I paused a second, reliving the examination in my mind before continuing. "It was the abdomen that was striking, her belly was distended, bowel sounds diminished, and there was diffuse, rebound tenderness. Yet, she moved easily around the bed, not like a patient with pancreatitis or an intestinal perforation."

"Ted?" the chief asked, his pencil momentarily stilled an inch above from his legal pad. "So far there's nothing to suggest gastroenteritis, such as diarrhea or abdominal cramping, and the tenderness could have been modified by the prednisone medication. Am I correct?"

The chief and I were on the same wavelength after only a few minutes of my presentation.

❖ ❖ ❖

I was the only resident or perhaps the only person in the world who called him "chief." He was Dr. Rhimes to everyone else. Even to Mrs. Rhimes. The "chief" moniker was a reaction to my early but brief Catholic school background with the despised formality of giving the "yes, Father," "yes, Sister" and "yes, ma'am and yes, sir," over and over to every adult who crossed my path.

I was the only child in my neighborhood and perhaps the only child in history expelled from a parochial school to obtain discipline at the public school. It started when Sister Ruth and Sister Eugenia ganged up on me after the fire incident wanting to see if I had matches in my pocket. It was the same Sister

Ruth who had piqued my interest in science, as I struggled to understand the physics behind the magnitude of pain she could inflict with a twelve-inch wooden ruler held at the tip—striking at the speed of sound on your arm or ear or scalp with just a flick of her thin wrist. Sister Eugenia was more conventional with her pointer used as a spear or a club; and her hands—hands the size of Texas, exploding from her rustling black habit, the color of a coal mountain, that were on top of you quicker than an eye-blink, twisting you skyward by your shoulder and shirt collar.

❖ ❖ ❖

"Chief, the rebound abdominal tenderness was worrisome especially with Mrs. Schmidt taking prednisone."

The chief nodded in agreement and asked for the results of the laboratory tests and abdominal X-rays. But I interrupted him, because I needed to tell him about the ecchymoses, the bruises, the blue monstrosities that dotted Mrs. Schmidt's belly and back. It was the reason I was there.

# THREE

"Ted, the new lupus patient of Dr. Rosenthal, appears ill and her husband is upset, and not at us, but at his wife." Nurse Sophie stopped me when I arrived to see Mrs. Schmidt. "He's the kind of lug who looks like he might turn violent at a moment's notice. I'll hang around when you go in there to see her." With that, I think Sophie was trying to be helpful not questioning my manhood.

"Thanks Sophie, for your assistance. It's my good fortune to have you around. Here, let me check your muscles." It wasn't easy for us to save our monkey business for after working hours. Adroitly dancing backwards, Sophie stayed out of reach. She was quick and nimble, even after a long day of running up and down the hospital floors. A knee-length, belted white cotton skirt topped with a thick blue apron rested inches below her knees and led down to laced pristine, rubber-soled-white-polished shoes that would also be at home on a tennis court.

All the rooms on this side of 3 General Medicine (3GM) were the same: single beds centered in the middle, the ceiling high enough for kite flying, and in spite of windows sealed shut, the floors hosted a permanent draft that turned unadorned toes blue.

I knew these rooms like the well-thumbed medical textbooks piled high on my bedside table. I could navigate through them in the dark. And I have. The john on the right, sink with antiseptic for my hands on the left, one plastic chair placed under the no-smoking poster, and immediately above the bed, protruding from the white painted plaster, like the snout of the Creature from the Black Lagoon, were the suction and oxygen tubes and call buttons and electrical outlets that made it a hospital room and not a slum rental.

Mr. Schmidt was sitting quietly in the corner, eyes fixed on me, no response to my "good afternoon." His perfunctory handshake came late. One of those meaty guys with hefty, wide shoulders and a belly to match, hands that blocked the sun, a prominent jaw, and an occasional flicker of a smile, more like a facial tic that under no circumstances would be considered charming. If he provided you with a service, you'd pay his bill without a complaint. And you would mark "excellent" across the board on the printed job-rating form he shoved at you before you even checked his work.

"Mr. Schmidt, good to meet you," I said. "I'll need privacy for the medical examination, especially the pelvic exam." I held the door open and shooed him out.

The tender bruises on Mrs. Schmidt's belly and back were the size of a large fist and resembled abstract paintings spotted with blue tints. The lighter edges merged into the pink of normal flesh. I tried to keep my face straight when I spotted them, but still Mrs. Schmidt caught my surprise.

"Every once in a while Tim gets violent, but he's a good man most of the time. He's a good father and breadwinner, but I worry about his temper now when I'm ill. He doesn't handle a sick wife very well."

I nodded my head. That was what they all said; a gentle, kind man—until he's not. I encountered that too often, and I've tried to stay non-judgmental about the volatile nature of certain couplings.

Mrs. Schmidt had aged well. Marriage at seventeen and pregnant soon after, she once was the local beauty and that spark persisted in spite of illness. Medium height, well-proportioned, no need for nips and tucks, hair bleached regularly at the neighborhood beauty emporium, combed carefully, make-up in place, even now her pride insisting on powder and rouge before being driven to the hospital. Prednisone medication added a flush and a trace of puffiness to her face. Neither were distracting. She had been hoping for good health, romance and gaiety in her life, but then so do we all. The confident Tim had been an aggressive suitor and impossible for a young girl to refuse.

I drew the blood for the laboratory tests—her veins were generous,—always a good prognostic sign. I marked the tubes "URGENT," started an intravenous line using the same needle and infused 5 percent glucose in half normal saline, taped the line and needle carefully to her skin, and phoned X-ray scheduling for a stat abdominal obstructive series.

I was ready for the mister. The worn white plastic chairs scattered in the hallway for the families to wile away the hours offered little comfort, especially when you were oversized with gargantuan feet in constant threat of being trampled by the food and snack and medicine carts, the wheelchairs, the pink-and-white-gowned candy stripers, everybody on a mission, everyone in a hurry. The scrambling back-and-forth with no one yielding the right of way, matched the chaos of downtown Marshall Field's on a Christmas holiday afternoon. Nobody silent in spite of the Be Quiet signs placed every ten feet at eye level, with the 1940s, blue-eyed, white-capped nurse, Jayne Mansfield clone, so deliciously stern with her shushing index finger pressed tight against generous-sized ruby-colored lips. I couldn't estimate the number of times I'd stared at that poster and shouted my devotion to her.

Betty sat upright in bed and Mr. Schmidt and I stood next to one another. She had become first name ill. "I'll telephone Dr. Rosenthal as soon as the laboratory tests are available and after I review the X-rays with our radiologist," I explained. "But I want the surgery team to examine you." I pointed to Betty and spoke confidently. Surgery consultation was mandatory and not really open for discussion. "Dr. Raul, the surgery resident, is on his way. There's a possibility of vasculitis, a frequent occurrence in lupus that could require further studies and possibly surgery."

"Mr. Schmidt—Tim," I turned to him—first names create a team mentality—and asked, "How hard did you hit Betty? Do you think that might be causing some of her symptoms?" My expression was bland, my question meant to be routine. I wanted to assess Tim's response to my perhaps-unexpected loaded query.

Betty and Tim shared glances, a scene reflecting brooding warfare that would never be amenable to change. Tim turned to me; I was on shaky ground. I'm usually non-confrontational at work.

"Doctor, we had a minor disagreement while I was drinking. I pushed Betty. I feel terribly sorry about it." He paused again. His blue eyes danced around the room like a Harley-Davidson hog weaving through rush-hour traffic. "Betty bruises easily. You know that's due to her lupus. I don't think we should talk about that. You look like a competent doctor. Just help Dr. Rosenthal and the good Lord to get my wife better."

I liked his contriteness, although we both knew the bruises weren't from pushing or minor disagreements. We shook hands again, united in helping Betty.

"Tim, pushing and shoving aren't tolerated in the hospital, and never solve any problems—well you know that," and I left the room to talk to Sophie, comfortable that Tim's anger had subsided, but first showing Betty how to use the call button.

❖ ❖ ❖

"Chief, I spoke to Dr. Rosenthal about Betty and told him the preliminary laboratory tests were reassuring. There was mild anemia, the white blood cell count was low, typical for lupus and suggesting no infection, and the platelet count was 80,000/cubic millimeter, also low, but not likely to cause bleeding. The X-rays revealed no free air under the diaphragm and non-specific ileus, making a gut perforation unlikely. The chest X-ray was normal."

# FOUR

Dr. Raul knew the importance of the blood sugar, the plasma volume, renal perfusion, sodium and potassium levels, all the specifics that only the medical residents and none of the other surgeons-in-training were familiar with. Lupus to Raul was not an alien life-form visiting from Alpha Centauri.

Caustic and sharp-tongued and usually with good reason, Raul suffered fools and non-surgeons poorly. In spite of that, we got along. We even drank beer together. The problems I had with him were his social skills, movie-star face and professional-soccer player physique. He spoke literate English and fluent, precise Spanish, exciting the young Latina staff, who shook their impossibly trim pelvises in ecstasy over this man when he shouted orders. Furthering my resentment was his cosmopolitan bearing, which thrilled Nurse Sophie.

"Go for it," clapping me on the back after he had thoroughly examined Betty and reviewed the X-rays. "Mrs. Schmidt, you're in good hands, with Dr. Ted here," providing her with a theatrical wink. "We don't think you have a surgical abdomen." Turning to me, he said, "Treat the inflammation, the medical problems first, and let's monitor the response." His words sounded very much like an internist.

I started one gram of intravenous prednisone in a small amount of saline solution attached piggyback to Betty's intravenous line after discussion with Dr. Rosenthal. Peritonitis and vasculitis caused by lupus inflammation were the probable diagnoses, and they likely explained Betty's rebound abdominal tenderness.

Raul and I would return in several hours and reassess her.

Betty thanked me for the attention.

"I feel better already, Doctor, and I know I'm in good hands with you. Please watch out for me." Our hands touched. I nodded my head and offered a smile meant to be reassuring.

"I promise I'll be here for you, Betty, and I always keep my promises. After all, I'm young and sincere, a budding physician since a tender age, and I'm smart, handsome, and modest too. I want you to get well and get home soon."

She smiled for the first time that day.

❖ ❖ ❖

Dr. Handler was our family doctor back then. Making a house call in the neighborhood, he spotted me and my co-conspirators start a fire in the alley, mixing the fall leaves with yellowed newspapers and dried twigs and featuring a battered doll borrowed from a little sister. It was the kind of doll with a once-white, now-spotted, dirty-gray cloth belly that bleated plaintively when bent at the waist. Its shrill sob entertained us for reasons known only to God, as we readied our weekly Joan of Arc reenactment. We were never lemonade-stand entrepreneurs or hopscotch enthusiasts.

"Ted, if you or your friends catch on fire, don't run," Dr. Handler lectured, his manicured fingers planted on my shoulder. My buddies had turned their backs and slinked into nearby backyards.

"Running will fan the blaze and make the fire spread. Stop and roll around in the dirt. That will smother the flames. Do you understand what I'm saying?" I nodded yes to the doctor's question. But he wanted more, and asked me to repeat his advice out loud. And I did.

Satisfied, he rewarded me with his genuine smile, the one flashed to the grown-ups after our fevers had broken, and walked on. Dr. Handler was a realist and I had read his concern, knowing that yelling at me about my innately acquired pyromania would be unproductive.

Right then, I understood that doctors were about more than administering shots and delivering bad news. Thoughts about my future shifted from soldiering and piracy to the medical care of the needy and beautiful.

Several years later, at a time when my father no longer could help me with the rigors of algebra and prime numbers, a time when futures were being discussed, a father-and-son time, he said to me, "*Dr. Ted*. Don't those two words sound right? *Dr. Ted*," he said again, as if peering into my future. "You'd be the first doctor in the family. I'd be very proud." Since I was too old for him to tousle my hair, he clasped his hands in mock prayer and bowed a little like a Japanese businessman, and laughed that warm laugh of his. He never mentioned it again, but his "*Dr. Ted*" stayed with me like the Bible stories of childhood filled with angels and miracles.

❖ ❖ ❖

I explained our plans and diagnosis to Tim and suggested that he head home soon. "The situation is under control," I said, spoken to him with the know-it-all smugness unique to the medical profession, but at the same time I wanted to dismiss this wife-beater and get him away from Betty.

Sophie's shift was over. Maria Amoroso, the evening head nurse, was brought up-to-date about Betty. Almost all the evening and night nurses at our institution were Filipina. Some were better trained than others. Maria was the best, and tonight she was working both the evening and night shift, back to back. We were covered. The usual midnight to 8 a.m. crew was scary. Who in their right mind would work those crazy hours? Their en masse departure in the morning, frantically shading themselves from the early sunlight with cupped hands snug on their foreheads, awkwardly seeking out shadows and stumbling over cracks in the sidewalk, became the inspiration for zombie movies.

Sophie hugged me. "I'll see you tomorrow. Thanks for seeing Betty Schmidt so quickly and thanks for the good care you provide."

Dr. Raul, having completed his note in Betty's chart, also gave Sophie a hug, and she repeated the same endearments to him.

"*Adios*, precious Sophia," Raul told her, kissing her hand too long. Sophie smiled at him, but blew me a kiss, mollifying my jealousy.

❖ ❖ ❖

We reevaluated Betty in two hours. I arrived before Raul. Surgeons were never on time. But Raul got a pass. Tim had left for the cafeteria; it was getting late and he hadn't eaten for almost a day. I had wolfed down the green Jell-O mold fifteen minutes before, found in abundance in the no-wait salad line, bits of something trapped inside, possibly peaches, topped with whipped cream and accompanied by saltines. The latter were free, and although I was feeling less than sated, the Jell-O combined with the recurring bumps of epinephrine stimulation during the day's on-call adventures kept my appetite in check.

The medical-on-duty resident—and that was me—stems the deluge, and the beeper never stops. The last phone call forwarded to me from the page operator just minutes ago was the daughter of a recently discharged patient: "Hello, Doctor, I wonder if we could chat about my mother's illness," she asked.

Well, "*chat*," was not an everyday word in my vocabulary, and since I didn't know her mother, and it was late, and after I ascertained there was no real emergency, I declined to "chat" and referred the daughter to her mother's attending doctor.

"My supervisor?" I responded to the daughter's query. "You want to complain to my supervisor?" Not incredulously expressed; after all, I was placed on earth to be helpful, or more accurately "somewhat" helpful, no blind number was tendered this lady. Mrs. Gail needed to earn her pay and retirement benefits, so let the daughter complain to her, and I provided Mrs. Gail's daytime phone, as those digits flowed from my memory banks quicker than the gravity-driven slide of the Jell-O concoction.

❖ ❖ ❖

Betty asked about lupus, and its cause, for which I knew little. "An autoimmune disease," I said knowingly, as if that explained things. "For some reason you're making antibodies against yourself and that's invoking inflammation." "*For some reason*" was the equivalent of the definitive "*because*" answer offered to children needing explanations for their awkward queries.

From under her pillow came photographs of her children. School pictures, I think, posed faces of beautiful children, an older daughter held in Betty's right hand and a son in the other, their hair too neatly combed and their posture too formal for their wry grins.

"Doctor, will they get lupus, too?" Betty asked.

"I don't think so," I said. "There's some familial tendency for lupus, but it's not very great. Plan on full and productive lives for them, so if you haven't started saving for their college educations, you'd better start now. And Harvard is expensive. But that one with the smile,"—pointing to the daughter, "*Celeste age ten*" handwritten in pencil on the bottom white sliver of the photograph—"looks like acting school material, and Hollywood success will be right around the corner."

We laughed.

"Betty, tell me more about you. No need for both Dr. Raul and me to push on your stomach and lean you forward to listen to your lungs. We'll do that together when he gets here."

"St. Xavier High School!" I repeated her response. "You went there? The miles I traveled to beg those girls to cooperate in the backseat of our automobiles—Betty, sorry I missed you, but you would probably have just kept on walking, head held high, too many suitors, and too lovely to pay attention to smart-alecks like me. Plus, the transfer of grease from my hair onto those Catholic schoolgirls' pristine white blouses was a turnoff."

"Doctor," she smiled—"you're nice, and thanks for taking charge of my care. You know what you're doing and thanks for the explanations. I would have said hello to you if you had driven by; too bad I'm old enough to be your aunt or older sister. I'll have Tim bring more photographs of my children tomorrow posing with their 'young' mother. I agree with you, they're beautiful kids. I'm not so sure about their mom, you can decide that for yourself," Betty said smiling again—"but it's the children who turn heads. When I get out of here, we'll have you over for coffee so you can meet them. And Tim can be sociable, especially when at home on a weekend and after a beer or two. You can tell us about medical school and why you became a doctor."

The knock on the door was Raul. What was that all about? Surgeons burst in, they didn't knock.

❖ ❖ ❖

Raul and I agreed that Betty had improved. The abdominal pain had lessened, she was afebrile and the bowel sounds remained audible. Her chest was clear, and she freely moved around the bed.

Betty thanked us for the attention and asked to be left alone. She needed sleep. "Send my husband home. He'll be less upset tomorrow and I'll feel safer, sometimes he scares me."

Tim was noncommittal when I brought him up-to-date and angry when I asked him to say goodbye to Betty with me around. I would telephone him in the morning and report on Betty's condition.

"You're basically a prick, Doctor. Stop telling me when I can see my wife." His angry mouth near my face, his fists clenched, violence was programmed in his genes.

"Tim, go home," I ordered, while we stood chest to chest. "You don't want me to call Security to escort you to your car. Get some sleep yourself. We'll all be happier in the morning."

He maintained his glare, moved back an inch, sneering at the idea that Security could handle the likes of him and instead of departing, sat down in the rear of Betty's room near the door, defying me to do anything about it.

I should have called Security, but Tim looked more tired than dangerous and Betty had fallen asleep.

Finishing my rounds, I talked to the students on my team about our shared patients, ambled off to the on-call resident room, and collapsed on the starch-encrusted hospital sheet covering one of the beds. My wash-and-wear tan cotton slacks and blue, long-sleeved shirt, with only a few green Jell-O splotches on the front would look considerably worse in the morning. Lord knows what would be on the back. I had once awakened with a "*please perform a stat rectal exam on this oaf*" sign attached.

I was surrounded by the smell of the hundreds of previous bodies who had spent interrupted nights in this cheerless, windowless room with a bathroom plucked *in toto* from nearby Comiskey Park immediately after a sold-out game.

Its stench was authentic stadium washroom, with the dripping faucets mysteriously becoming noisier as the night progressed. Thoughts of Tim Schmidt's anger and Betty's fears circled through my conscience, but the sleep of the on-call resident slammed down its steel curtain.

# FIVE

My recurring dream pictured a hospital room with the magnetic poster board across from the bed stating: *Today is* ***Wednesday****. Your nurse is* ***Mae West****. We are here to serve you promptly.*

All falsehoods, the nurses seldom came running, especially if you were in pain, and they looked more like William Claude Dukenfield, aka W. C. Fields, than Miss West. Anyway, today was Tuesday.

The cleaning person floated into view, her back to me, rubbing the bedside table and water glasses with the same gray cotton rag used to scrub the toilet bowl. The telephone rang, loud and incessant like an explosion from a clock radio on a dreary Monday morning.

Hidden in the dark shadows, near the minuscule closet, stuffed with the ill-fitting paper gowns and slippers, I unobtrusively observed the hospital routine. The room, identical to all the others in my dreams, was as expansive as a convention hall, the walls painted matte black to absorb joy, the large windows shuttered, hosting the same patient, her features vaguely familiar, someone from early childhood perhaps, a teacher, an across-the-street neighbor, the grocery store lady. I was unsure. Lying still in a too-large bed, she was covered with a quilted black comforter, the rim of a neatly folded white sheet setting off her gaunt face. An orderly pushed through the swinging doors, his face immobile and stark, maneuvering an empty stretcher, walking goose steps, ready to transport the patient to an alternate universe.

I moved in a dreamlike glide, legs floating in midair, toward the clanging black telephone atop the flat-topped, black steel bedside table.

Nurse Sophie joined me, always helpful, her blouse open, smiling her special smile, reserved only for me, and I guess Dr. Raul. Floating together, our bodies touched, as we headed toward the earsplitting sound of the telephone. The scene, so fascinating in its quietude except for the ringing, as Nurse Sophie and I together recited, "*The bell tolling for someone, perchance even for me.*" I turned toward her and buttoned her blouse, my hands inadvertently stroking her chest, provoking promises of intriguing favors, as she cupped my fingers with hers.

I snatched the phone receiver. The patient's skeletal hands clawed at my coat and arms, fighting for the handset. "Let go, dear, it's the chief offering me a position in his laboratory for next year and thanking me for my vigilance in enforcing high-quality hospital standards," I said, stopping to scold the cleaning person, who was rubbing my INTMED 3 badge with the multipurpose scrub rag that had recently shined the commode.

The chief spoke to me in falsetto.

"Dr. Ted, a Code-One on 3GM, are you awake, Doctor? Please answer me."

Why was the chief telling me this? What about the research offer?

It was Gertrude, the nighttime page operator, not the chief, not even Mrs. Gail, or Nurse Sophie whose breasts were replaced by the saliva-soaked pillowcase brushing my face.

"Oh, shit, Gertrude," I said. "I was deep asleep and I thought the chief was trying to reach me. What do you want?"

"A Code-One, Doctor, on 3GM," she repeated.

In thickened utterance, I acknowledged the location and assured Gertrude I was alert and awake, then rolled out of bed and stared at the radioactive glow of the dot numbers in my otherwise black watch dial with the worn leather strap indented into my wrist. For a nominal price, the watch provided the correct time to the second and removed hair from my forearm.

Still dazed, I was now able to button my white coat and rush out the door, shaking my head to banish the cobwebs, no time to brush my teeth, tongue furiously working the edges of my mouth removing the nighttime grunge. I'd kill for a stick or two of Wrigley's Spearmint gum or even a few tiny rectangles of Dentyne. My hands brushed my hair back and forth into a semblance of order, the on-call pager nestled in my pocket near my pelvis, intensely vibrating, also announcing the Code-One and stoking my Sophie fantasies that were fueling my erection.

I sang my special Code-One mantra, spewing it by rote after so many past repetitions. "Don't let it be someone I know. Don't make it unexpected. It's okay if it's a false alarm." Wishes seldom granted. I was ardently anti-geriatric, as I added: "Let it be someone who's had a full life, someone who's experienced a multitude of pleasures and disappointments, someone older than sixty-five."

In charge of these Code-Ones daily for two successive weeks when I rotated through the cardiology month, I couldn't use the john without anticipating the telltale vibration and ring of the Code-One beeper. Everyone else on the resuscitation team would be miffed about finding a healthy person or someone postictal or post-syncopal, but breathing, and with normal heart function. No cardiac or pulmonary arrest, no life-or-death drama to play out, no struggling patient lying at an odd angle, eyes beginning to dull, surrounded by medical and nursing staff positioning a hard wooden board under their spine to augment the force of our chest compressions and mute the charge of the electrical stimulator. No suction pump siphoning the debris pooling in the mouth and nose, booming in the background as we shouted instructions to one another.

Giddy with pleasure when I found a healthy person, I would dance around the bed. No electrical shocks to the left chest or epinephrine inserted directly into heart muscle from a syringe and needle the length of the Eiffel Tower, followed by head-shaking, downcast eyes and the solemn pronouncement of death. We were the Spanish Inquisition resurrected again in hospitals in the late 1950s and early 1960s.

Young enough to run up the stairs at full speed, mouth less gritty, alertness returning, asleep for only three hours, it's still a struggle to awaken in the middle of dream sleep, but I never begrudged the sudden return to consciousness. I wanted to be the person at the bedside. That's why I was a doctor.

I knew in my heart that this Code-One was for Betty Schmidt, although my rational mind said it couldn't be. A stat page from Maria that Betty had worsened or spiked a fever was understandable, but not a Code-One.

Maria Amaroso and the anesthesiologist stood in the hall, palms vertical, directing me to slow down. In charge of Code-Ones, I didn't like to be told what to do, but I stopped and listened, my feet jitterbugging, ready to make life-and-death decisions.

"It's Betty Schmidt," Maria spoke first. There were cogent reasons for me being a pessimist. Three lousy words, enough to sink my heart, make breathing painful, my mind filled with expositions: heart attack, pulmonary embolus, massive hemorrhage, but the most compelling of all, a vision of Tim doing something terrible to his wife.

The anesthesiologist said, "She's cold, chilling already, probably dead for an hour. Please tell me you don't want me to intubate her."

Betty was distinctly still, at peace, her body bisecting the bed, nothing out of order, gown in place, eyes shut, motionless, cold and lifeless like a portraiture sketched by an amateur. The three of us, heads down, lips moving, offered a silent prayer. Maria and I crossed ourselves just as the crash cart with the other members of the Code-One team arrived, pushing into the room, cardiac-paddle ready, the door banging back and forth, way too loud for so late at night, the room instantly filled with white-clothed emergency doctors and technicians brandishing their breathing bags and intravenous bottles.

"Go back to sleep," I told them. "Thanks for rushing here."

But before they left, I asked: "Do you see anything unusual here?" Sure it was late and they were tired, their eyes still, wanting to move on after hearing their reprieve, but that didn't stop me.

"Did you ever see a coded patient lie so goddamn neat like this, in such a pre-Raphaelite pose? Like Ophelia, lying at her wake for chrissakes! This patient didn't fight for her life or even struggle to tell the nurse that she was short of breath or experiencing chest pain."

My associates stared at me, burdened with incomprehension fueled by tiredness, and wondering who in hell Ophelia was?

"Lupus patients don't die quietly in their sleep" My finger pointed toward Betty and then at them. "She should have pressed the call button for Maria," I said, as I mimicked the compression of the call bulb with my thumb and forefinger held in front of my face. "And she should have screamed. Don't you see there's something's wrong here." My harangue gradually wound down into a whisper.

A few noncommittal nods and pats on my shoulder, no one really upset with this death but me. And I was left alone with my ward, the person I'd promised to take care of, help, make better. Now she was a corpse.

"Thanks, Dr. Ted for your expert assistance and for being there when it mattered," I said to myself, but loud enough for the words to reverberate through the room.

"Did you touch anything? Did you tidy-up?" I asked Maria, now sitting quietly at her desk. Her chores were just beginning—the telephone calls to the morgue, to the funeral home, to the administrators, to the housekeepers. The voluminous paperwork meant for the bureaucracy of the dead: the hospital, the city, the county, the state, demanding to know the time and why, but not offering a speck of sympathy.

And there always was another patient sitting by a phone waiting for admission to the soon-to-be empty room. No one informing them: "Oh, by the way, someone died in that bed just a few hours ago."

"No," Maria said. "I'm so sorry Dr. Ted." And she was saddened, her heart joining mine at the lowest level of despair. "We had an emergency, an admission requiring surgery that took all my time, but I told Mrs. Schmidt to press the call button if she needed anything. When I returned to check her vital signs, this was how I found her."

"Where was Tim—Mr. Schmidt—when all this happened?" I persisted, standing in her vision, trying to sort out the events. I knew I should have called Security and walked Tim to the parking garage instead of leaving him in Betty's room.

"I saw him leave after I found Betty dead. I only saw his back as he went into the elevator. I didn't see anything else. I'm really sorry, Dr. Ted."

It's one of our unwritten rules. You don't leave an abusive spouse like Tim alone with your charge.

I had ignored it. What a loser I was. What was it about me or my training that had failed Betty? I should have looked in on her again before I fell asleep. I should have sent Tim home. I should have done a lot of things differently. My helplessness added rage to my sorrow.

# SIX

If you have a loved one in the hospital and the phone rings late at night, don't answer.

"Tim, its Dr. Ted. Are you awake? Are you sitting down? I have bad news." The words hung in the air with a weight of their own. I've participated in these conversations countless times, and I'm never sure what to expect.

I was sitting at the nurses' station. It was quiet there. Bad news was quiet.

"Betty died. I just came from her room. I'm sorry. This was so unexpected. I don't know what went wrong. I don't think there was anything we could have done differently. Again, I'm sorry. The autopsy may give us some answers."

It was late, I was exhausted and my words rushed out like a teenager driving a souped-up eight-cylinder hot rod on a deserted highway. Saddened and angry about Betty, I was unsure how to approach Tim. Was he the grieving widower or a murderer?

"Doctor, I'm devastated. Betty's dead? I just left her, this is unbelievable." Tim spoke slowly, his voice steady, a whisper. "Thanks for calling, but I don't need to think about anything and I can speak for everybody in the family. We don't want an autopsy. I don't believe in cutting up a dead person. She had lupus, a terrible disease. I wouldn't wish it on anyone. This is terrible news—just awful. I loved her."

"Tim, sorry to interrupt, but whenever there is an unexpected death, especially in a new hospital admission, the county coroner will insist on an autopsy. We have no choice about this."

It wasn't exactly true.

I'd contact the coroner at a reasonable hour. They didn't appreciate phone calls in the middle of the night. It was always a game with the coroner. Subtlety works, but Mrs. Schmidt's bruises and sudden demise were such that we and they couldn't afford to miss a homicide.

"Tim, I'm sorry about the delay the autopsy will cause, but I'll make sure everything will be done as promptly as possible and I'll call you with the results. Please accept my sincerest and deepest condolences about Betty. This wasn't how we planned it, and I'm devastated."

"Doctor, I know you heard me. Don't you dare hang up. We don't want an autopsy. Cutting up a loved one—my wife—is against everything we—I—believe in."

"Sorry, Tim, I have to do the right thing. Betty shouldn't have died. There's something the matter here and we need explanations."

I gently hung up the phone after the silence.

Dr. Rosenthal was never at his best at this time of the morning, and that wouldn't be helped by the type of news I was delivering.

Twelve rings, and still his "Dr. Rosenthal," sounded like the Mandarin version of his name. "Shel, it's Ted. Sorry to awaken you, but Mrs. Schmidt died a short while ago. I know, I know, I couldn't believe it either. The whole team was there for her arrest and she wasn't revivable." I didn't tell Shel that poor Mrs. Schmidt was cold by the time I arrived.

"Sorry, Shel, I have no explanation for her death. The admission electrocardiogram was okay, there was no ischemia and no arrhythmia, and her electrolytes were normal."

After an eternity, I asked, "Shel, are you there?"

"Shit, Ted, how did this happen? Why wasn't I told that she was so sick? Why wasn't she transferred to the intensive care unit where she could have been monitored more diligently? Where were the floor nurses? Why didn't you request a private-duty nurse? Has anyone told the family?"

This was Shel at his best, shifting the blame with one question after another.

"Shel, I feel as bad as you do. I don't know what we could have done differently. I've informed Mr. Schmidt and I'll call the coroner's office about an autopsy. Do you have any suspicion of foul play from Tim?"

Again a pause and then, "I heard you Ted, I'm not that asleep. Tim, a murderer? I don't think so. I've known the two of them for some time. Was he drinking last night? Ted, it would be best if you don't even go that way. That's big trouble."

I gave Shel Tim's phone number and then hung up.

❖ ❖ ❖

"Chief, I spoke to the coroner and he said quote, 'Fuck its six a.m., do whatever you want. Call me if you find something worrisome and forward the final report.' I also spoke with Jane, the hospital lawyer."

I had placed the ball in the chief's court so when Dr. Rosenthal and Tim Schmidt finally got through Mrs. Gail and started yelling at him, he'd be prepared.

# SEVEN

Jane, the hospital lawyer, did the practical stuff. When we had once worried about being sued after botching an emergency procedure on a semi-comatose, mentally challenged adolescent, we called Jane.

Jane was on loan from a planet of blue-eyed citizens with golden strands of wheat-colored, shiny straight hair that swayed with every graceful breeze. Tall, athletic—WASP athletic: tennis, golf, field hockey, unlikely wrestling, but one could always hope—and the whitest, straightest teeth this side of the Hudson. Descended from a prominent old-line family, she stuck out as a beautiful alien in this predominantly Jewish hospital with its black, blue-collar workers and the occasional *goy* troublemaker like me. And since all was right in our world, and good things do come to pass, Jane and Howard were betrothed.

"Good morning, Ted" Jane was disgustingly bright at 6:15 a.m. "Is everything okay? What's going on this early and beautiful morning?"

You can understand my adoration for dear Jane.

Jane agreed that an autopsy was justified on poor Mrs. Schmidt.

"Is there anything I can do? Call the coroner, telephone Mr. Schmidt, whatever?" she asked. I declined assistance. She wished me "the best" and asked to "please keep her informed."

❖ ❖ ❖

When our residency started, the first year medical residents attended a getting-to-know-one-another party at Jane's parents' house in the posh North Shore. The music, alcohol and exquisite finger sandwiches were far too sophisticated for us. Howard introduced himself to Jane's parents by requesting cold beer rather than one of the six choices of imported wine, along with permission to dance with their daughter.

It was weeks later when Jane told me the two of them wandered into the library, sitting down at the grand Steinway centered in the book-lined room designed for the Sun King. Shoulders rubbed together on the long black wooden piano bench, windows opened to the garden. The roses were in bloom, the deep red color of the flowers, almost magenta, peeking into view, taking in the spectrum of human foibles. Howard, tall, posture erect, played "The Girl with the Flaxen Hair," his long fingers caressing the melody, his eyes meeting Jane's. The rose perfume saturated the air, the splendor of their youth, the beer and wine, the glorious music, Debussy himself would have been enchanted with the concatenation of two handsome souls capturing each other's hearts at that precise moment in space and time.

# EIGHT

"Ted, how many cases of lupus have you seen?" the chief said, opening his tobacco pouch, letting the aroma spread across the desk for a moment. The filled, half-bent briar was his solace.

"Lupus patients die young. The years of unchecked inflammation, the ravages of the prednisone, the narrowed coronary arteries, the clotting propensity, they all lead to premature heart disease. If Mrs. Schmidt didn't die of a myocardial infarction, she died of coronary ischemia causing an arrhythmia, or she suffered a pulmonary embolus. There won't be any surprises, although I'd be interested in the extent of the vasculitis. You should have asked Dr. Rosenthal about the need for an autopsy. I know about his difficulty awakening, but he's an experienced doctor. Or you could have called me, especially when the husband was so upset about the procedure."

*Puff, puff*, the downward flame of the lighter working perfectly, the aromatic smell of the premium tobacco mixture and the pause in our discussion offered by his smoking timeout, and his enjoyment of the splendid respite, all gently defused our colloquy.

"What were you looking for with the autopsy? Were there new signs of violence?"

I shrugged my shoulders, not ready to voice my belief that Betty had been suffocated by her husband. "Chief, the spousal abuse surely aggravated the bowel symptoms. Those injuries cause damage," I answered, hoping instead, as the chief suggested that we'd find a straightforward cause for Betty's death—a major pulmonary embolus for instance, something quick and painless that would have been untreatable in the middle of the night. That wouldn't offer me much comfort, but it would alleviate a considerable portion of my guilt.

"Ted, you were the doctor on the scene and I respect your decision-making and I'll support it." The chief was calm and reassuring, his eyes following the pipe smoke twisting upward before returning to mine.

"You made the right choice by coming here this morning. Go back to work. I'm also concerned about the bruises that were present on the patient. I'll handle Mr. Schmidt and Dr. Rosenthal. Refer any calls from the Schmidt family to me, and I'll transfer them back to Mrs. Gail. She'll know what to do," he said, flashing me a brief smile, enjoying the minor levity.

"I'll telephone Dr. Wendle in Pathology," he added. "I'll ask her to perform the autopsy herself, and you, Ted, please, please keep me informed about subsequent happenings." His face softening, reading my tension.

"These unexpected deaths," he continued, "well of course any death, you know what I mean, gets us in our heart, right here." The chief gently poked himself in the chest for emphasis, not spilling a shred of tobacco—"and in our psyche" not needing to point to his brain, while I nodded in affirmation. "It affects us deep to the core. We can't help it, that's what makes us human. But we must learn from these sad encounters and move on. I think the right word is '*perspective*.' It's a lousy word, I know, and it becomes too much a part of our lives. Events, like last night with Betty Schmidt, will be frequent occurrences. Let them reside quietly."

His advice came from the heart, his brief smile was my dismissal, and he returned to his papers, his head down, visibly aging each time I visited.

# NINE

Three General Medicine was bustling. Students and residents prodded the patients, their heads down in concentration, hands pushing abdomens—right upper quadrant for liver and gallbladder, LUQ for spleen and turn of the colon—then came the "*how're you doing*?" The orderlies shuttled patients back and forth, the phlebotomists blood sucked, the nurses placed medications in white paper cups, vital signs were recorded—multiply the chaos by admissions, or deaths, or transfers, or discharges, or being shuttled to surgery, and the disarray mimicked Soldier Field after a go-ahead touchdown against the Green Bay Packers.

The surgical team crowded in front of me with their wrinkled scrub uniforms. Dr. Fineglass was the exception; and no Dr. Raul, who was most likely in the operating room removing bullets lodged deep in a vital organ or stitching a knife wound while displaying his charms to the OR nurses.

"Dr. Ted, how's Mrs. Schmidt? Dr. Raul is busy in surgery," Fineglass, the satrap, the second in charge, asked his question delivered as if he were astride a military horse surveying the carnage.

"She's dead, iron fingers, and probably with multiple perforations that you missed. I paged you all night. Where were you?" My words spewed into his face, my index finger slammed into his chest. Everyone has to let go of tension, me especially since Betty's death. I didn't mind getting Fineglass's dander up, because I disliked him with a passion. He had nothing to do with Betty's demise, even if it turned out we missed an intestinal perforation.

The morning-after call is never an easy one and Fineglass always appeared too composed, too unperturbed. He didn't dress like a surgeon either, more like a board-meeting attendee. His pristine nametag featured sparkles and funny animal stickers stuck to it so children would like him. They didn't.

Fineglass didn't like to get his hands dirty or wet. He once asked the operator to page a student to draw blood from a patient lying right in front of us. "Asshole!" I yelled at him as soon as we reached the hallway. "Don't ever call somebody to perform scut work when one of us is around. Never!" I cancelled the page, drew the blood and tubed it to the laboratory. Fineglass was too quick on his feet for the gloves I threw to hit him.

"Fineglass, you look lovely this morning. I didn't know that clip-on ties came in such lustrous colors. Red and white polka dots, how wonderful—did it catch measles?"

I pointed to his blindingly white and pristine shoes—I would've paid a million dollars to be able to pour piss or iodine on them—and I danced around the monstrosities singing the "Buster Brown" radio jingle for the edification of his team and for that matter, all of 3GM: *"I got shoes. You got shoes. Why, everybody's got to have shoes! And there's only one kinda shoe for Fineglass—good ol Buster Brown Shoes!"*

I must have insulted the prick, or perhaps he wasn't a music aficionado, or maybe his shoes were Florsheim's or Thom McAn's, because within minutes, I was paged for 2-6000, Mrs. Gail's number. She picked up immediately. "Four p.m., and be here on time! What in God's name did you sing to the surgeons? And what do you have against the handsome and polite Dr. Fineglass?"

❖ ❖ ❖

Fineglass was engaged to a medical resident who was one year behind me in her training. Estelle and I worked together one night, one of those nights with too many admissions and too many ill people. While performing a lumbar puncture on an uncooperative woman, Estelle needed my help soothing the patient and the handling of the laboratory and culture tubes.

Our hands and bodies politely touched in the tiny room as I opened vials, unwrapped syringes, and gently crooned to the patient, who requested divine assistance for a getaway vehicle. Truth was, I was always willing to hang around Estelle. I'd admire her beauty and try out my cache of recently acquired locker-room jokes.

"An old man goes to a doctor for his annual physical and his wife tags along. The nurse tells him they need a stool sample, a urine sample, and a semen sample. Being very hard of hearing, the old man yells at his wife: 'What the heck do they want?' The wife yells back, her mouth inches from his ear: 'They want your underwear.'"

Not to be outdone, Estelle responded, gloved hands, mask loose over her mouth and nose while capably performing the lumbar puncture: "What do you call a one-legged woman? she queried. "Eileen," she answered after my shoulder shrug.

"And what do you call a one-legged Asian woman?" she asked again. "Irene," she said, not waiting for my reply.

And so it went.

It was late, we were tired and it seemed funny at the time, and we were young.

Count the number of women you can pine for and exchange jokes with. And her ready laugh spilled out with enjoyment and zeal. Her auburn hair was pinned tight in a bun behind her graceful neck—I'd give up a vacation day to plant a wet kiss there.

It was 2:15 a.m., each medical floor had big, round, white ceramic-faced, electric clocks with long sweeping second hands sitting high over the chief nurses' desks. We needed the correct time for the TOD, the time of death. We could err with our medical diagnosis, but not the TOD.

I remembered the time. But then again it's always that time. It has nothing to do with numerology. That's the moment in our diurnal rhythm earmarked for infidelity. Heightened by the adrenaline rush after a death or a life saved, the touching, the kissing, the screwing, the too many young doctors, nurses, students, too much excitement, too much proximity, it was all there and it all began then.

They were not affairs or trysts. They weren't even one-nighters. There was no planning and there were no explanations. We talked about them as "roll-a-rounds," and I guess that's what they were. Offering no framework for a meaningful relationship, but like a first date or the first French kiss, it was impossible to forget the edgy passion that erupted from thin air.

The lumbar puncture was completed, the antibiotic hung in a free flowing intravenous line, the spinal fluid tubes sent to the laboratory for culture, cell count and chemistries—and the patient quiet and breathing peacefully. The latter was more easily accomplished once the needle was removed from her back. The seconds ticked loud over our shoulders; there was no other noise at that time of night, just the *tick-tick* and no one but us to hear it.

Opposites attract. That's the gospel. But the funny thing was, Estelle and I, we're not opposites at all. We're both the wise guys pushing against authority, making waves, not to make a name for ourselves, well, yes that also, but mainly to try to help somebody, or change the system for the better.

Estelle reached out and edged her warm hand down my shirt, the top button undone from the arduous day on call, my tie knotted at half mast. She cradled my spindly gold cross hanging from its long, filigreed chain, her fingertips quick and light like the scurrying of a trapped spider. I kept the cross inconspicuous, lying far down on my chest, flattened by my clothes. It had belonged to my father—religion, like politics, was private, he preached. But sometimes during the heat of a Code-One, it flew out, as if testing its wings. Estelle centered the cross over my mouth, then surrounded it with her tongue and lips, pressing it tight until I could taste the alchemy of warmth and woman.

We locked the door of the examining room. It was where we performed procedures and where we sat families down for the bad news recitations—the place you never want to be. Tonight, the activity would be more catholic. Estelle pulled up her starched, white cotton doctor's skirt, wriggled her panties down with her hands and legs, and stretched supine across the flat examining table. The back of her long, slender legs stuck to the white paper cover, rustling and crunching with her stirring, and, as if touched by a magician, her skin and clothes became silk.

The thoroughness of the fuck, after our long, busy schedule-induced abstinence, and the sudden release of our neglected ejaculatory muscles stretched way too full, pleased us with repetitive contractions, bringing out laughter—joyous, primitive, involuntary, and boisterous laughter.

"Wait a minute," she said, as she stood and pushed me onto the examining stool, moving me away until my back hit the wall, and fellatio when you're excited takes little time. Ignore the notion about a refractory period when you're young and aroused at 2:15 a.m.

She wiped herself with the brown paper hand towels stacked in tandem in the nickel-colored metal dispensers overhanging the sink, climbed back onto the examining table, and announced, "Your turn Doctor," directing my face to where she wanted attention. Sated and ready to dream the dream of the contented, I instead was pulled into her secret world of warmth and slippery splendor, tasting darkness and confection, heeding her cries of "higher" and "harder."

"Good going, stud," she finally said, pulling her skirt down and panties up, juggling them in place, patting them straight, smoothing her hair to neatness with practiced hand, hunting her reflection in the full-length mirror on the far wall, pleased with the results, mirrors being Estelle's friend. Standing closer than Siamese twins, our skin and wrinkled clothes perfumed with the scent of arousal and hospital antiseptic, I readied for our postcoital kiss to be mixed with a multitude of sweet murmurings and a gentle hug, perhaps even to linger for a few minutes, a perfect finale after our screwing and feast. Instead I heard: "If you ever tell anyone about tonight, I'll cut your cock off." Her hand smack in front of my face, her fingers scissoring up and down, and then she walked out.

Three weeks later and I'm told she was engaged to Fineglass. I saw the diamond rock on her fourth finger as we were shoved together in the crowded elevator heading up to the medical floors. Eyes forward and fixed on the battered metal door, I whispered from the corner of my mouth: "*How could you? He wears argyle socks, white bucks, and today his fish tie is wrinkled...*"

"I told you "higher" and "harder," but did you listen?" and she exited past me on the third floor, giving my shoulder a no-nonsense shove.

❖ ❖ ❖

The chief let me off easy, probably running low on tobacco and ready for his Scotch. It was already after 4 p.m. I promised to be civil to the surgeons, agreeing they were an integral part of the hospital team and entitled to respect.

"Chief, thanks for your patience and I'll try to control my temper."

*Wait until I see that snitch, Fineglass. I'll accidentally break one of his fingers during a conciliatory handshake. The surgery morbidity statistics will improve and my spirits will get back on track.*

Leaving the chief's office, I had the opportunity to thank Mrs. Gail for my Thanksgiving Day duty assignment.

"The holiday dinner will be celebrated right here at the hospital cafeteria, the food's delicious, the line moves smartly, and maybe you'll consider gracing my day by being my guest." I said. "The stuffing is exquisite, you know, it's really quite delicious."

Having piqued her interest, Mrs. Gail remained unsure whether I was pulling her generous leg or not.

"It's shipped in direct from Los Angeles," I said. She looked up, intrigued with any culinary knowledge I might possess. Her eyebrows raised, her mouth pursed in surprise, her typing stopped, hands in midair, the Remington quiet. "It's simmered in the La Brea Tar Pits and that wonderful burnt taste stays with you for weeks. I'll try to save you some if you can't get away," and with that I turned and departed.

# TEN

The morgue resided in the depths of the hospital. Press the red Sub-B button on the elevator panel, turn left to the thick doors blocking the exit that featured an inoperative *MUST RING BELL TO ENTER* buzzer. The *Abbott and Costello Meet Frankenstein* soundtrack played in the background as the doors creaked open with concerted pushing. Finally, an ANATOMICAL PATHOLOGY sign over a door with frosted glass that should have been printed with the words reading "temporary resting place," or simply "the morgue, we screwed up and that's why your beloved is here before he or she will be buried for eternity."

I stuck with my charges until the end. They became part of my life and then too often they ended in the subbasement. Cancer, heart attacks, strokes, there were too many ailments and too few answers. I'd like to never come down to this place, but that would make me less of a doctor. We've learned through our years of training that sometimes there's only a spark between life and death. But not in the morgue—here they're always dead.

Dr. Wendle was Wendy to me. Nobody knew her first name. The first openly gay person I knew. It was shocking for the time, when her Naomi came with her to hospital functions, and although public displays of affection between them were uncommon, it was clear that these two upstanding, normal-appearing people were partners—and not in the law firm sort of way. Maybe they'd inherited a genetic defect.

"Dr. Ted, my hard-working buddy, you must have been on call again," Wendy said. We laughed, we were friends, but the levity was short-lived, Betty was down here.

Short, attractive, with all-seeing brown eyes, this hardworking, middle-aged doctor was nationally known for her skills in defining different types of lung injury. Dr. Wendle was also a gloriously outspoken Diogenes. Not nasty, not devious, straightforward and polite, her usual affirmations went thusly: "What you're saying, Doctor, may be very important, but this is why the patient expired."

For the first time, I actually said what I had been thinking since Betty's death. And I said it to Wendy, rather than pussyfooting around it the way I had when I talked to the chief.

"The patient had lupus and an acute abdomen, but I think her husband straddled her and suffocated her with something. Her death was too quiet, too unexpected, her posture too unruffled; it was as if the funeral director had already paid a visit, applied his cosmetic magic, and tidied up. There were old bruises on the body and a long history of spousal abuse." The latter would get Wendy's attention she abhorred violence.

"Asphyxiation is hard to detect unless there's a struggle," she said. "Let's take a look." And with that, we entered the dissection room, which was kept at near-freezing temperatures to slow the decay. Only one table was occupied. It was constructed of cold, shiny stainless steel and placed high off the floor, brilliant fluorescent lights overhead eerily illuminating the body, scattering odd elongated shadows over the rubber mats and cement floor. Water trickled from every faucet, the soothing sound offsetting the business-like roar of the circular saw separating bone and flesh. Bright enough for a movie shoot, the morgue was only absent cameras and extras.

The diffident morgue attendant, head down, all business, prepared Betty for the autopsy. This was not the place for weak stomachs. Betty was supine, nude of course. Blood mottled around her back and sides, gravity worked quickly in the dead. The ugly blue layered above the pink flesh. Tim Schmidt was correct. No one wants an autopsy performed on their loved one.

Thick rubber gloves stretching up to her mid forearms, Wendy searched Betty's face, inspected her nose, touched here and looked there, angling Betty's head for more light, her eyes sometimes less than an inch from Betty's face.

"I don't see evidence of facial trauma," she told me. "It could be that there was no suffocation, or the patient was deeply asleep and asphyxia came quickly.

There's nothing obvious," she said. She wasn't going to look again. "Don't call me. I'll telephone you with the gross findings later or come down this afternoon if you're able to get away. The microscopic sections from the organs will be ready in a few days."

I was dismissed. Wendy would turn up her music when she was finished with me. The Ramsey Lewis melodies would linger longer than the formalin and body odors of the anatomical pathology laboratory. There was no place for me to kneel so I sat down on a small stool with four wheels, lowered my head, and spoke to the soul of Betty Schmidt.

*"Betty, I believe that when good people die, they travel toward a better place. Every time someone says a good thing or thinks a good thought about you, you get closer and closer to your journey's end. If there was foul play, I'll get to the bottom of it. I'll pray for you.* Pax tibi, *rest in peace."*

I paused. My litany wasn't finished. I needed another moment to gather more thoughts. *"Betty, it's me again. I'm going to wait for the autopsy results; then we'll talk and discuss our plans."*

# ELEVEN

Morning report, a tradition at teaching hospitals, was the forum where we discussed new admissions from the previous day and reviewed follow-up information about patient outcomes from prior days. The chief medical resident, an honorary appointee made by the chief, served as the referee. It was a good place to obtain second opinions and it offered a quality check for our patient care. Sometimes there were too many opinions, and discussions often mimicked transcripts from a *Three Stooges* short.

Morning report could make or break your reputation. Internal medicine training was a battle. You wouldn't think so by looking at the pale and bespectacled faces fidgeting around the messy conference table, but underneath the residents' mild-mannered repose dwelled rapier wits, supported with a depth of arcane knowledge. Sometimes the medical residents were just stupid and loud.

Food and coffee were served—not enough for everyone, but as an incentive to arrive on time. There was a misconception about doctors in training and their body habitus. We were the opposite of gaunt, making up for missed meals with the free ice cream, jelly doughnuts, bacon, and mystery meat gulped down between emergencies in the late evenings. And since Mrs. B headed home at sundown or 5 p.m., whichever came earlier, even the doctors not on call and their friends, dates, wives, children, and their children's friends helped themselves to the largesse. Mashed potatoes with brown gravy pooled precisely in the center of the tasteless white mush and diced Del Monte pineapple bits floating in heavy syrup were the side dishes offered with everything. As for exercise, we were way too tired to do anything extracurricular, and we waddled around, ten flabby pounds over our fighting weight.

My team talked about our admissions and I deflected criticism about our decision making. There were times when the students or residents shed tears from the gibes graciously offered by their contemporaries, who saved their more vicious salvos for the weak and dull. I happened to be a master of morning report.

I talked about Mrs. Schmidt, leaving out her demise until the end, and then everyone, and rightfully so was appalled. My adversaries, suddenly awake and in attack mode, questioned my decision-making, not allowing this get-even opportunity to escape them.

Fists pounding in palms, I was told that we should have operated; or not given corticosteroids so quickly or that we administered either too much or not enough; that we should have performed a stat abdominal angiogram or not—the suggestions running the gamut of medical testing and therapeutics.

Quiet and humble, I promised to report back in a day or two when autopsy information became available, and yes, maybe transferring Betty to the ICU for closer monitoring would have saved her life. Tim wouldn't have been able to suffocate anyone in the busy and monitored ICU. The nurses were tougher there; one nasty look or word from him and Security would have escorted him out.

Chuck, our reigning chief resident, notebook in hand, sidled up to me at the end of the hour. "Ted, that Schmidt patient was fascinating. Would you spend about fifteen minutes talking about lupus and sudden death on Friday? We'll learn from the discussion. I'll also invite Dr. Trillup, you know him, the lupus expert from the university, to speak to us. He'll offer wisdom about Mrs. Schmidt."

"No," I responded.

I was going to walk away, but I have an inexplicable soft spot in my heart for Chuck, the chief resident. Whenever I heard the name "Chuck," the "chief resident" descriptor spewed out of my mouth with no additional thought. If that bothered Chuck, the chief resident, I don't know. I don't think so. He was quiet and good-mannered and his smile remained sincere.

I disliked him for other reasons too.

He was one of those lucky guys who excelled at everything. A champion wrestler on the college team, who, and this stuck in my craw the most, when he quickly pinned you, helped you up and thanked you for the excellent match. And he meant it! It was impossible to adequately describe the dislike I had for a gracious winner.

In spite of his smarts—and he was very smart, in addition to being neat and fair and honest, and available for all of our disputes—he was clueless. Some turd would tell him that he couldn't be on call that day because his grandmother had died for the fifth time that year and Chuck, the chief resident, would remove him from the schedule and commence an avalanche of on-call adjustments. It proved to be so easy that I wouldn't take advantage of it. Between the schedule changes he concocted, and Mrs. Gail's nastiness, I was on call every holiday and every Saturday of the year. My only free day was Christmas. I would shamelessly play the religious card and not work that day, even if it fell on a Saturday.

Internal medicine was filled with Jewish doctors. Jews weren't welcomed in the surgery specialties. They weren't nimble with their hands, and since they were so smart, worked so hard, and had no vices such as imbibing beers with the urologists, they automatically migrated into internal medicine, the thinking man's specialty. It was in their genes.

Being Polish, I was the special case. We sat around discussing who was going to do what for the high holidays of Rosh Hashanah and Yom Kippur, and I would be so unnaturally quiet, my associates would say, "*Sorry Ted, we forgot you're not Jewish.*" "You're forgiven," I would quickly reply. "How about buying me a beer to make up for your rudeness?"

When I was the only non-Jew at the cafeteria table crammed with my contemporaries, I would acquire a pious expression, lower my head, authoritatively tap a water glass with a metal tablespoon, and command: "Let's pray together. Bow your heads for chrissakes, we're all children of Abraham!" And I'd prattle on for minutes, always wondering to myself if Ray Morales, the Filipino vascular surgeon, or Bob Linn, the Chinese cardiologist, were also children of Abraham. I thanked God for the beautiful day, or the rain, the food, the tasteless coffee, the runny, scrambled eggs, Thelma the page operator with the hearing deficit,

Mrs. B with her goddamn chamomile tea, Mrs. Gail and her charm—until a heretic, someone clearly not ready for sainthood, would say, "Shut the fuck up already, I'm hungry!"

I was prepared to talk about Mrs. Schmidt again. I wanted to research it, and if Chuck, the chief resident, could persuade Dr. Kenneth Trillup to travel to our institution and talk about lupus and Betty's untimely death, that would benefit all of us. The good lupus doctor would immediately know something was amiss.

# TWELVE

Howard was happy, not just content but happy. Every time we traveled to Maddie's on Madison Street, the bar with the lap-dancing, big-busted girls and eight ounces of stale beer for five dollars, he'd tell me the pleasures life offered: Jane, the practice of medicine, his fellowship training plans, and of course, me sitting right next to him.

Maddie's owner was a patient of ours, and he had instructed the girls to provide extra friction. Attractive and businesslike, the young ladies were pleased to see us, well at least for a few minutes, telling us about their medical problems before leaving for richer pastures.

Maddie's was an old time tavern and meeting place. Built before Prohibition, but not successful until the cachet of getting high on moonshine became popular, it was the place to be seen on a Saturday night in the twenties and thirties, when it was okay to rub elbows with gangsters, sport stars and politicians. The influential people had left decades ago, but the city's downtown was moving west, gentrification was encroaching, and the clientele becoming upscale once more. The mixture of the pretty girls, the businesspeople, and the blue-collar crowd wanting a safe place to drink, provided a fascinating machismo, a guys' place with sports and politics, and of course, the girls.

The dark mahogany paneling covered with grime and plans gone wrong was being renovated, scraped, sanded smooth and stained, and the Byzantine-influenced white-tile marble floor was cleaned and patched, and one of these days Howard and I wouldn't be admitted without sporting a tie and receiving a nod from the boss. Smiling, efficient bartenders nodded in agreement with our lame arguments and supported our idea about lap-dancing punch tickets, but get out of line with one of the girls and a club appeared quicker than your dollars disappearing from the bar top.

You wouldn't think a tavern was a place for contemplation. But the beers and the darkness and the noise isolated us, cocoon like, with our thoughts remaining private. That night with Estelle, how does nature allow something so brief to linger so long? And Betty, always Betty! Her illness had tried my expertise—a young and vital patient, an uncommon medical problem, a right-on treatment regimen—it was so hard to fathom what went wrong, and then to live with the consequences.

Howard would use the quiet moments to badger me about my lack of plans for next year. Some of the Jewish medical groups had doubts about employing *goyim*, and no private practice tenders were forthcoming. Of course, it could have been because of my lousy personality. Further training in an academic center began to seem appealing, but I needed laboratory experience. Herb Rhoban, the head of hematology and my mentor, as well as Dr. Rhimes, extolled the time they spent performing basic research. I tasted the excitement their investigations generated, as I began to understand their stellar accomplishments.

"Howard, we're medicine's Corsican Brothers: clinicians, researchers, troublemakers, thinkers, planners, 'one for all, and all for one.'" Mixing metaphors with the best of them, we toasted each other with the mugs of beer, pleased with our businesslike deliberations.

No time to ponder my future the last night we'd visited Maddie's. The jerk sitting next to me had spilled beer on his neighbors and blamed me. In places like this, if you have too much fun, bad things happen, like a Friday night baseball game at Comiskey Park, when the inebriated teenagers, tired of the ball game, began to search for more excitement than a stolen base or a passed ball.

Big Goon, his face marked with trouble and his mouth contorted with hate, told me that my elbow had hit his drinking arm, causing him to spill beer on his friends. Alcohol mellows some men; this guy's hackles became raised.

"Hey fellows, sorry about the spilt beer, but it really wasn't my fault, take my word for it. Remember please, the wisdom of Georg Wilhelm Friedrich

Hegel, the great German philosopher you're no doubt familiar with. He provided salient advice: 'The nature of humanity is to impel men to agree with one another.'" Hegel should occupy this sorry-looking group and their stunted neurons for awhile.

Big Goon, not pacified, pushed my arm, a no-no, and asked me who was going to pay for the cleaning. This guy was a combination Neanderthal and Nephilim, the latter being giants who had inhabited Canaan according to the book of Numbers.

"You must be confusing me with someone who gives a shit," I said with a smile and I turned away to talk to Howard. If Big Goon's brain was TWA airplane mileage, he'd get as far as Oak Park.

We had had enough beer, the bubbles had disappeared a long time ago, and we paid the bar bill and departed. The night was cool and crisp and perfect until Big Goon accompanied by several henchmen burst out of Maddie's and rushed toward me. Before he could utter one evil word, I clocked him. There's never a reason to wait around for the shoving and the cussing and the spittle. For better or worse get on with it.

I hit him in synergy with my anger for having to partake in this deed. Un-doctor-like, I delivered a right hand to his nose, resulting in a satisfying *crunch*, straight to the target, the shortest distance between two places, my knees slightly flexed, feet moving up on my toes, my fist making a twist to the left after contact, then back in place ready to launch another punch.

The goon's nose hemorrhaged. The blood supply to the nose is generous, as are pain fibers, and both were now fully activated, making him grab his face, when I unleashed my left hand. I throw combinations; my boxing lessons took. I hit him in the right eye. Head bent over in pain, he was energetic enough to lift his leg, trying to kick me. I grabbed his foot, and lifted it skyward while pushing toward him with enough force to put him on his back with a *thud*. This meeting of the working-class miscreant on alcohol versus the doctor-in-training continued in my favor.

My epinephrine level was high enough to arouse a dozen of the recently deceased, and I kicked him with my plain-toed faux cordovans, assuredly not with the efficacy of work boots, but if you keep kicking at the same site, the pain increases exponentially. His buddies kept away, because I was a demon and because this guy was a *schmuck*. Maybe they knew justice was being dished out. Howard had snatched the bouncer's club, keeping it visible at shoulder height, also discouraging mob action. He returned it to the bouncer-observer when the show was over, placed an arm around me, and suggested we move on.

Howard drove back to the hospital. My hands were sore. A boxer will often fracture the fifth knuckle because of the impact. All of my fingers were tender, but they moved well. X-rays weren't needed, ice packs would suffice, and a few more beers would reduce the discomfort.

# THIRTEEN

Dr. Wendle informed me that Betty Schmidt had myocarditis, inflammation of the heart muscle. No pulmonary embolus or heart attack or bowel perforation, the more usual causes of death were found. Several areas of bowel ischemia caused by vasculitis accounted for the abdominal pain. The bruises produced by Tim were superficial and hadn't contributed to Betty's demise.

"I relayed this information to your chief of medicine. He called me about the patient. I'm signing her out as death due to an arrhythmia, secondary to lupus inflammation of the heart," Wendy said, handing me the autopsy report.

More frustrated than angry, I remained standing in her compact office, not wanting to sit in her proffered chair, and complained. "You describe here," I scanned the now official report—"a smidgen of vasculitis, a little heart inflammation, the latter not even bad enough to cause heart failure. You don't really know the terminal event. Just write the cause of death was uncertain and that asphyxiation can't be excluded. Arrhythmia is only your best guess. Yes, don't deny it it's just your guess," I said, not pointing at her, but gripping the ledge of her desk, as if I were hanging on for dear life on an Alpine mountain cliff. For the first time I let my ire surface, my voice becoming strident. "This lady was murdered and you're dancing around the issue."

That caught Wendy's attention, but she was never displeased by disagreement.

"Ted, if I wrote 'asphyxiation' for this lady based on your reasoning, I would have to write that about everyone who comes down here. Sorry." Wendy spoke softly and gently, aware of my concerns. "There's room for argument, but I think there's enough inflammation in the heart for me to support a cardiac death."

She turned back to her music, now filling the background. The Modern Jazz Quartet had replaced Ramsey Lewis. Milt Jackson's vibraphone pulsated in my ear—Willow Weep for Me mellowing our world, "*listen to my plea/hear me willow and weep for me*" as Wendy patiently waited for additional comments or complaints.

What was Betty going to think when I relayed this news to her?

❖ ❖ ❖

The chief warned me about calling Tim Schmidt, but I had promised Tim I'd telephone him about the autopsy. And I wanted to stir things up.

He answered immediately. Just a curt "hello," and when I told him about the autopsy report, he uttered softly and barely audibly, but with the resolve of a bandit requesting a victim's wallet after placing a long knife on his neck: "You cut Betty up to find out she died of lupus? I could have told you that! Doctor, I won't forget your screw up and the pain you've caused us. Never! Watch your back!"

The slamming noise of the phone rattled my tympanic membrane.

❖ ❖ ❖

It was time to telephone Stan Glicke, the most prominent criminal defense attorney in the city. He had been my patient on several occasions and more would be in the offing. Stan suffered from a unique medical problem that none of the other residents wanted to treat, or even talk to him about. They would page me to insert his intravenous lines and perform the venipunctures, hesitant to touch him in spite of doubling up on surgical gloves and donning paper masks.

Stan experienced recurrent infections I only discussed with him and his psychiatrist—illnesses brought on by sexual depravity. And he reveled in it. Otherwise, he was a fine, upstanding citizen, charming and brilliant.

Stan suffered from diabetes mellitus that needed constant monitoring and frequent insulin injections. Kidneys, eyes and heart functioned normally because he took good care of himself, carefully checking his blood sugars, eating sparingly, exercising regularly, and faithfully visiting his endocrinologist. Yet, in spite of his excellent medical etiquette, his penis remained limp. Go figure. It was not because of lack of lascivious thoughts.

The blood vessels down there weren't dilating normally, or maybe the sacral autonomic plexus malfunctioned, or the corpus spongiosum couldn't fill properly, or something like that. Diabetes was the pits for male happiness.

After successfully representing a client, which happened often, his name splashed on the front pages of our three daily newspapers, Stan would treat himself to a respite in the Caribbean and entertain a slew of young women for X-rated activities, none of which included the missionary position or any position requiring an erection. He would return with gonorrhea in his bloodstream and mouth and every other orifice. And gonorrhea of the oral and nasal pharynx was never a pretty sight.

Intravenous penicillin would lower the fever and soothe the sores after a few days. Inability to swallow for that time contributed to a sizeable weight loss, and his diabetes control would improve.

"Why didn't you take the penicillin tablets I gave you?" I asked, which always prompted a lame excuse. On this occasion, he had donated the pills to one of the girls because she had a cold. "Doctor, I wouldn't want to love a woman with snot crusted across her nose and sputum erupting between her lovely lips like Mount Vesuvius every few minutes, now, would I?" Stan related this to me in his best lawyerly voice and assumed I would agree with him.

And he was entitled to the best medical care without criticism of his exploits, no matter how unsavory. I reminded my associates to remain nonjudgmental and preach preventive medicine. But it was I who performed the examinations, started the IVs, wrote the medication orders, played nurse, doctor, and confidant.

Stan's secretary found him immediately.

"Stan, I know this sounds as if I'm confabulating, but I want to discuss a hospital homicide with a police officer. I want someone who'll listen to me and tell me I'm not being foolish. Do you know anyone like that?"

"*Boychik,* a hospital homicide mystery, it sounds as if there's money to be made, especially if it goes to trial. Be sure to let me in on the ground floor. Call

Sergeant George Esposito at the Third Police District in the Homicide office. I knew him when he was working Organized Crime. He was too damn effective there, so they transferred him to Homicide. Tell me a little about the case and then give me a few hours' head start and I'll telephone him first. Okay?"

I could picture Stan at his desk, feet up, Montblanc pen twirling around his index finger, an Egyptian cotton white shirt, 1,000-ply or 100 stitches per inch, enough white to blind a stadium of Reverend Moon newlyweds, while he carefully listened to every word I spoke. Because hidden behind those ordinary brown eyes and bland expression was a brain filled with more connections than a nuclear power plant.

Stan always looked good in spite of his afflictions. Fifty-two years old, and he had been that age for the two and a half years I had known him, and why not? It was a good age and easy to remember unless you played pinochle. Custom-made everything, hospital pj's, jeans, three button suits, white shirts with French cuffs, and red silk ties: "Red like bull," he said, the latter depicting his courtroom jousts.

"Stan, it was my patient, an ordinary patient, ill, not life-threatening ill, but she died in the middle of the night, never even ringing for the nurse. The husband, a wife-beater, was left alone with her, and nothing was found on autopsy that explained her death, well, anyway, that's the official interpretation. I think the spouse smothered her."

"Ted, stop! What kind of murder case could it be if the autopsy didn't show anything? That's a big problem. Call me back if she was rich or if there's a contested big-time will, or the killer spouse is a movie star, and hey, Doc, I may be seeing you soon. "It's vacation time and I need a parcel of exquisite loving," he said. "How about joining me? My treat, of course, since you're my personal physician, it'll be a business expense, and I suspect you're a fun guy."

"Thanks for the kind offer, Stan, but you know I can't get away, what with my work schedule and all." Our visions of paradise differed greatly.

# FOURTEEN

The police station resided less than a mile from the hospital, two stories high, faux prairie school but with graffiti. Close to Chinatown, it should have featured a pagoda instead of a leaky roof. It was Sunday, and in spite of the rising crime rate, my car was the only one parked in the visitors' section. Maybe if more citizens talked to our guardians, the city would be safer.

The desk sergeant pointed out my name printed in pencil on his handwritten list and waved me up a flight of worn stairs with a flick of his beefy hand. Not a stairway to heaven, yet the passageway wafted an aura of spirituality, as if by traveling skyward, step by step on the hardwood stairs worn smooth from the footprints of serial killers, lawmen, burglars, liars, and the naïve such as me, one would find enlightenment.

Sergeant George Esposito's cubicle was located as promised, his desk as scarred as mine, but his to-do list featured the names of unsolved murder victims. Mine had the deli takeout menu, and the Rice Krispies Treats recipe, the one I crave, the one spiked with miniature marshmallows and dark chocolate stars. The knock on the plastic side panel was greeted by a middle-aged face, hardened by years of serving and protecting. But a hint of tolerance and a suggestion of a smile shined through the toughness, dampening the unease I always felt when around law enforcers—a firm handshake, and a formal greeting and this policeman became my public confessor.

George Esposito could have starred in the movies, the older and wiser partner, the ex-soldier with the chiseled face and buzz haircut, who gets it at the end protecting the star, rather than sitting on 22nd Street fighting urban crime. Only later did I see photographs of a younger army MP, assigned to that job because he'd enlisted to become a helicopter pilot. There was inquisitiveness about him, perhaps newspaper reporter genes dwelling inside his protoplasm. Maybe he was gathering material for a soon-to-be bestseller book describing the city's murders.

The coffee was familiar, likely purchased from the same jobber employed by Mrs. B, the cup clean with no sharp edges, still wet on the outside from the cold water rinsing, the dark liquid hot with steam spiraling upward, mixing with the stale air. We sipped the coffee, measuring one another. George leaned back in his chair, arms behind his neck and listened to my story without interruption. I finished by telling the sergeant I had promised Betty Schmidt I would take care of her.

Our clothing tastes were similar, wash-and-wear brown sport coat, and khaki-colored pants of shiny synthetic material, the same Sears on-sale merchandise, his everyday clothes and my dress-ups for special occasions such as these. We were the same size, extra-large, "husky" or "solid" as they used to say, but even without gel I had better hair.

"We don't get too many doctors coming here," he said. "I don't remember a homicide like you described taking place in a hospital room, at least where we were able to prove it's a homicide when the autopsy showed no signs of foul play. I'm right, aren't I Doctor, your own pathologist doesn't mention homicide? Sitting here on an afternoon off presumably wasn't your first choice for recreation, although I appreciate your desire for justice." The sergeant spoke with avuncular concern, but he also seemed worried about my sanity.

The fugitive posters lining the wall with the ALIVE or DEAD reminders were the only decorations. No personal photographs or multicolored Crayola scribbles of bunnies and squirrels from nursery school-age children pinned on the poster-boards or taped near the desks. Work was too precarious to expose laughing progeny and handsome wives to the creepy visitors.

"I see that you think this homicide-division detective is your public servant with a paucity of work to do," now his cynical side was emerging. "You like the word '*paucity*,' Doctor, even though we're all ignoramuses here, and you're thinking, Gee whiz, there aren't enough unsolved killings in our fair city to keep us busy. Maybe I'll manufacture a shit homicide case from what sounds like a routine death, especially for the good Sergeant Esposito. He's the guy with the empty in-basket. The same guy who sees his family too often."

He studied me some more. Not as if I was a jester or a troublemaker, but as if he was intrigued by my motives for being here. Stan's telephone call, I'm sure, had paved the way for the sergeant's patience.

"It's keeping you up at night this case, isn't it Doctor? Plus, there's your own private guilt about losing a patient," he continued, transforming into my psychiatrist. "The other thing that I've learned through the years, Doc, and believe you me, it's a lesson worth remembering—don't promise a woman anything."

Laughing loud, the sergeant pulled out his chair, stood up straight, stretching his torso high before offering me more coffee, while at the same time asking for more information.

I didn't laugh.

"Sergeant, listen to me again. Please, listen again for another minute," I said, pointing at him and directing him to sit down. I wanted his full attention.

"Say, for instance, you're assigned as a bodyguard." I looked at the sergeant and pointed to him again with my index finger. "You're the best, you're in charge." I nodded my head at him. "You've trained for this assignment your entire life. It doesn't matter who you're going to protect, it could be the governor or it could be just some nobody, but whoever it is, they need your skills.

"Something bad happens out of the blue. The guy you're protecting gets killed. Not an act of God, lightning doesn't streak down from the heavens and settle between his eyes, a piano doesn't tumble out from the third-floor window onto his skull. Somebody murders him, and you,"—I pointed to him again—"you could have stopped it. But you didn't."

I paused for a moment and repeated my lament.

"It really doesn't matter how it happened. You didn't stop it."

I had the sergeant's attention. The Sunday hollowness of the squad room made my voice carry, Charlton Heston as Moses on Mount Sinai, speaking to the masses but minus the clay tablets.

"Now what do you do?" I asked him. "No," I interrupted myself, "make it, what do *I* do?" I paused again. "It's too late to save Betty, but it's not too late for me to want justice. And I want justice."

"Doctor"—the sergeant laughed and pointed his index finger back to me; police believe in immediate retaliation—"I hear you. Great speech and performed without notes, not even one index card, well done. We're speaking the same language. I'm on your side. I'll tell you what to do, what'll we do, but give me more details, and first just a little more coffee."

The atmosphere changed when I told the sergeant the husband was Tim Schmidt. He stopped for a minute, his gaze directed into the void behind me, coffee cup carefully placed on his desk with two hands, centered on top of the remnants of a legal pad; then he looked at me, before speaking again. Any lightness had vanished.

"I'm sure there are quite a few Tim Schmidts, but there's one we keep track of. Insurance scams, money-lending, fake auto claims, that kind of thing, an occasional strong-arm job, but no murders that we can prove. Doc, if this guy you're talking about is the same Tim Schmidt we know, he's well-connected, if you know what I mean. He's tough and lives in a physical world, a world far different from the doctor and nurse stuff that you deal with. Tim Schmidt, the one I'm talking about, is as bad as they come."

George queried me about lupus and its prognosis and asked me to talk to Wendy again about the autopsy results. "Also, query Maria Amoroso once more about the whereabouts of Tim during the hours before Betty's death. And I'll check to see whether there was a hefty insurance policy on her, or if this is even the same Schmidt fellow we know about. I'll get back to you and let you know what we find."

I got up to leave, mission accomplished.

"Doc, as long as you're here, can you give me a pill for insomnia and something for my back pain?" He motioned for me to be seated, his palm up this time, wanting to complete his litany of requests. "How about something for nerves, so I don't yell at my wife and kids all the time, or better yet, how about something for my libido—hey, that would help me forget about my other complaints? Do they make a combination pill like that? And how about a note for a two-week vacation in Hawaii as treatment for depression and over-work.

"You know, Doc, doctors and the police share a lot in common. We observe people closely, and we're forced to make snap judgments and sometimes even quicker decisions. I like that you came here. We'll try to work together."

I've always felt a kinship with cops. They're physical people, doing something that matters. And I liked this guy. I knew I sounded like an idiot citizen reporting a UFO sighting or ghosts in the attic, but George had listened like a trained counselor and I was appreciative. I was finally doing something for Betty.

# FIFTEEN

Hematology rounds started with chalkboard presentations. We'd post the admission dates, the laboratory results, the patients' hospital course, and then hunch over microscopes reviewing blood smears and bone marrow aspirations before marching en masse to the patient rooms. We were a boisterous group, a conglomeration of medical residents and students infused with youthful enthusiasm, but having difficulty being quiet, me the senior resident, in charge. "Inside voices, please," I'd say. A disciplinarian, seriousness tight on my face, sometimes I would single out a miscreant, making an example of him, finger to my lips, loudly shushing him.

There were other things too that I insisted on that were meant to expand our horizons. Such an insular bunch we were; it was if our memory banks were missing a primary color. Just past our east windows was Lake Michigan, primal as an ocean rumbling into the entire length of the city. "Which one of the Great Lakes lies completely within the United States?" I'd ask. No one knew. Medical students shunned the slippery courses such as sociology and philosophy, but apparently geography also wasn't part of their catechism. Late Thursday afternoons, right after Journal Club, we read fiction—my choice—*Nine Stories* by J.D. Salinger featuring "A Perfect Day for Bananafish." Bananafish had nothing to do with muscle insertions, or innervations, but I shouldn't have been the sole aficionado of the masterful tale.

Herb Rhoban led our procession, smiling in the face of too-often gloomy news. Herb was an expert on platelets, the tiny particles in our circulation that assist with clotting. Understanding their maturation in the bone marrow and release into the bloodstream ready to seal gaps left by injury, comprised his life's work.

What was it about these unselfish platelets, so important in the grand scheme of maintaining one's health that they prompted the body to make antibodies against them in lupus patients like Betty? Herb and I discussed this worry over coffee in his office resplendent with diplomas and acclaims, the photographs featuring his winning smile, never caught unprepared, his teeth on display, white, straight, and sparkling.

Herb was also the go-to hematologist for much of the city. If you had a blood abnormality or enlarged lymph nodes, you saw him, or it was off to the Mayo Brothers. Tall and fit, almost too good-looking for a doctor, he was blessed with a shock of unkempt dark hair like Victor Mature in *Samson and Delilah*. He possessed a ready smile and a wiry frame, casually, but expensively dressed with creased wool slacks, not the wide-wale tan corduroy or khaki-colored pants that were de rigueur for the rest of academia; and his leather shoes had matching laces.

Herb's clinical skills allowed him the freedom to be upfront about his opinions and decisions. Never second-guessing himself, Herb made life easier for us probationers. He was never wishy washy. Aggressive about treating cancer, more so than many of us thought necessary, he'd tell the family: "I only know how to try everything possible to keep your mother alive. I don't recommend halfway measures." Sensing their hesitation, he'd offer names of other physicians employing gentler management.

Herb and I played tennis together. It was always wise to play aerobic sports with a doctor-in-training. It was better than life insurance. You never knew when cardiac resuscitation might come in handy when you were middle-aged, trying too hard, breathing short, and down 40-love. Herb circled around the court like a wounded pelican and had no second serve to speak of.

Hitting the top of the net or stroking the ball inches past the baseline to make myself lose, took considerable skill. I'd drop the racket in disgust, choreographed with a stare to the heavens and a sharp talk with the divinity. Herb would be ecstatic, another victory, and his opponent nearly half his age. But there was a quid pro quo for my adeptness. I became part of his team, his advisee, privy to his skills and knowledge. Herb encouraged me to work with him after acquiring basic laboratory skills at a university research laboratory.

Contrast the happy us, as we conducted our rounds on the moribund clientele sheltered in our depressing institution with the surfeit of ill-chosen prints and posters hanging on the sterile white walls. Selected by young, overpaid, smiley consultants, who'd never been ill a day in their lives, they featured the art of distorted Picasso women with imaginatively depicted bizarre dreams leaking from their skulls and expanding circumferentially to complete the canvas. Edvard Munch painted a series of men screaming against a blood red background, and we had copies of all of them, every damn one, and just in case you missed any, there was at least one print on every floor.

We gathered around Mrs. Stone's bed, adjusting the curtains around her, as if that would muffle our pronouncements. The spare hospital room was small, two beds, the other occupant politely feigning sleep. Hanging from the wall centered between them, the poster board stated that today was **Friday** and your nurse was **Gloria**. It also should have added that Nurse Gloria was never around.

The room was ominously dark, the grime-covered windows and the tattered blinds denied the late-afternoon sun entry into this part of the universe. Thin and faded starch-encrusted mattress sheets had a mixture of urine and iodine melancholy. Contributing to the surrealism was the housekeeper hanging around, her cupped hand funneling our wisdom to her ear, so she could disseminate the news.

"Everybody, this is Mrs. Stone," I said. "Mrs. Stone, you've met most of our team, and I know you've already met Dr. Rhoban."

Herb shook hands with Mrs. Stone, bowed slightly, and said, "Pleased to meet you," for the fourth time that week.

I presented Mrs. Stone's story of fever, weight loss, anemia, bone pain, and fatigue and reminded the team about her bone marrow slides, which we had reviewed less than an hour ago. I talked in code about the presence of sheets of plasma cells filling her marrow cavity, establishing the diagnosis of multiple myeloma, a fatal blood disorder.

"You remember Mrs. Stone's bone marrow with the monotony of all those 'P' cells," our personal cipher for the plasma cells. I nodded knowingly at everybody, while smiling at Mrs. Stone—it was as if I had favorably commented about her handsome husband's face shining from the photograph propped lengthwise on her bedside table, rather than announcing her death sentence. Everyone knew the significance of the "P" cells except Mrs. Stone.

Mrs. Stone lay deathly still, praying that her cooperation would make us more astute and kind, while thinking about her appointment in Samarra. I had told Herb about an abnormal physical finding, and he plunged his hands into Mrs. Stone's left supraclavicular space feeling the same mass I had discovered.

"Does anyone know what a Virchow's node is?" Herb asked the crowd, always the teacher.

We all knew what a Virchow's node was, having had it repeatedly taught to us in our training. But being well-rehearsed, we shook our heads negatively to please him.

"I thought at least one of you would know what that was. I'm really surprised about what they don't teach you nowadays in medical school. Pay attention to me and I'll provide you with a lot of information." He was smiling happily, standing even straighter if that were possible. His day, if not Mrs. Stone's, becoming a success. "I'll tell you outside what it means."

Virchow's nodes were abnormal lymph nodes buried behind the left clavicle usually indicating cancer metastasis arising from the gastrointestinal tract, especially the stomach. Mrs. Stone likely had another malignancy beside the multiple myeloma.

Herb told Mrs. Stone about her myeloma diagnosis and explained that treatment needed to be started right away. "We'll prescribe cyclophosphamide and intravenous and oral fluids and you'll feel much better soon. And this excellent doctor"—pointing to me—"will stop by later and explain your illness to you." A big, comforting smile, Herb was pleased with his treatment plan. If he were to become depressed with every cancer he diagnosed, he wouldn't be able to enjoy a personal life.

Herb neglected to mention the side effects of treatment: hair loss, nausea, anorexia, infections, and the dismal prognosis of multiple myeloma itself. Sometimes I thought, and I thought about it too often, wouldn't it be better if we just gathered in the cafeteria, gorged on the mystery food they dished up in huge quantities until we became immobile like bananafish and then slept the afternoon away?

"Telephone Mrs. Stone's private doctor and bring him up-to-date about the diagnosis," Herb said, pointing to me and adding under his breath, "*but what a prick he was to have missed the diagnosis for so long.*"

As far as I knew, there was no cure for multiple myeloma no matter when it was diagnosed.

"Arrange for a surgeon to biopsy the lymph node after we go to Radiology and review her X-rays. Schedule an upper GI barium series, and tell Mrs. Stone and her private doc how we plan on proceeding. Would you mind meeting with Mr. Stone later? Sit down with him and bring him up-to-date because he's been telephoning all day."

Next patient and so it went.

❖ ❖ ❖

Mr. Stone and I saw each other daily. Years older than the missus, he had made no plans for widowhood. A believer in details and repetition, he had missed his calling, he should have been an accountant, and much to his dismay, I could only offer him the uncertainties about myeloma outcomes.

"Always be optimistic, but also tidy up loose affairs," I said to him. "Statistics apply to groups and not to individuals as lovely as Mrs. Stone. Let's take it day by day." Medical babble comprised one of the darkest sides of our profession.

# SIXTEEN

The sergeant had parked his car in the no-parking zone in front of the hospital's entranceway and strolled past both the security guard and the front desk with a wave of his hand. Compare the blue-collar policeman with his degree in law enforcement earned at the city college after six exacting years of weekend and evening study, with the world-class MDs and scientists at this prestigious center of learning who were not allowed to even think about abandoning their expensive German cars near the front entrance. Where were our standards, that this guy, like a sports hero, turned the heads of everyone when Nobel Prize laureates from down the street were required to sign in, disclose their mother's maiden name, their first-grade teacher's waist size, and an explanation for their presence in our hallowed premises? The latter, spoken with their right hand resting diagonally over their hearts, and then, and only then were they allowed to glue on a square, blue-and-white stick-on visitors' badge.

I excused myself from Herb and our afternoon rounds and met the sergeant in the hospital cafeteria. His suit jacket spread wide, offering glimpses of the revolver handle and badge, and his asking for me by name awakened the cafeteria employees, many of them hoping that he was there to cuff me, facedown on the floor. Mrs. B, overwhelmed by the sergeant's casual authority, danced around the register to greet him, snubbing the patron waiting for her change with outstretched palm. No hassling of the sergeant for on-call coupons or even money at all for that matter. Chamomile tea with lemon was not mentioned.

"Oh, miss," the sergeant acknowledged Mrs. B, "the coffee is delicious, you must have brewed it yourself, and my, you have a lovely smile." A cheap display of flirtation for sure, but endearing himself to the blushing Mrs. B as she rushed over with a refill.

My Mr. Schmidt had shown up on the bad-boy police sheets. Domestic violence was the least of it. No convictions, but lots of court dates.

"He's muscle for the mob, organized crime, remember, I told you about that possibility. An insurance office in the neighborhood, but he doesn't sell many policies, and in those he does, he's listed as the beneficiary. It included one on his wife, a quarter of a million dollars, and without much of a premium. There's lots of traffic in his office with big, mean-looking guys walking in and out. No one sits down, rests their legs on an ottoman, and swaps sugar cookie recipes."

The sergeant rested his elbows on the table, reveling in his disclosures to me.

"Rumor has it that Tim likes to get personally involved with the rough stuff, and word on the street is, he's good at it. And he manages to go free every time." The sergeant stopped to take a long sip of the coffee. He savored the stuff, his sips of the java, like kisses, as he worked his tongue and lips in appreciation, the dark brew likely his substitute for cigarettes and alcohol. "The gambling and mob law enforcement guys would like to get something on him—anything—that's why I'm here. He did kill his wife didn't he?"

"George, I think so, but I can't get our pathologist to even hint at it in the final autopsy report. She said that Betty, Mrs. Schmidt, had too much generalized inflammation, especially involving the heart, to not list lupus as the cause of death, and the trauma Tim inflicted didn't contribute to her demise. I disagree with her interpretation, but I'm just a lowly medical resident. My status in the hospital hierarchy ranks a tad higher than that of a medical student and several steps below the valet people."

"My captain," George said, "wants to bring Tim in and question him about his wife's untimely death, the bruises found on her body, and ask him why a young woman should carry such a generous life insurance policy and see how he reacts. No mention of your name, of course. We'll tell him our visit originated from the coroner's office, part of a routine investigation."

George seemed to be speaking to an audience somewhere out there, his eyes never on me. Aware, most likely, of the trouble I had made for myself.

"Tim's a clever guy, and he'll put two and two together. So, watch your step. Doc, be careful. Be extra careful! I'll tell him that if he goes anywhere near the hospital, we'll dump him in the river. If he brings his lawyer with him, we'll just tell him to behave.

"Now help me find your pathologist. I have an appointment to see her and ask her more about the cause of death. I, too, want justice to be served."

We shook hands. This policeman was a good man, and I appreciated his effort, his interest in Betty Schmidt, and his advice about being careful; although not to worry about the latter, I could take care of myself.

I needed to return to hematology rounds. I sketched a map to the morgue for the sergeant, walked him to the elevator, pressed the Sub B button and wished him luck.

# SEVENTEEN

*She said at length, feeling the doctor's eyes,*
*I don't know what you do exactly when a person dies.*
~Edna St. Vincent Millay

## *Bill and Amy Tomczak*

Bill Tomczak, a young accountant for a downtown firm, suffered a myocardial infarction, a heart attack. There was a family history of heart disease, but Bill was fit, a non-smoker, a family man filled with pure thoughts and noble deeds, too nice to have anything bad happen to him.

Bill's cholesterol was elevated. Researchers across town were beginning to recognize cholesterol as a risk factor for coronary artery disease, and there was a buzz about the illness after President Eisenhower's heart attack in 1955 and the ministrations of Dr. Paul Dudley White. The buzz disappeared quickly. The president hadn't suffered enough. A year later, a robust-appearing Ike was reelected in a landslide.

Transferred to my floor, barely forty years old, Bill handled this untoward event well, offering us good cheer before and after we listened to his heart. He vowed to eat less, exercise more, and continue nurturing uncorrupted thoughts.

Mrs. Amy Tomczak, also known as "the attractive one," as in "eyes front, the attractive one is here," visited daily, sharing her gracious smile, splendid figure, and a box of freshly made crème-filled chocolate doughnuts with everyone at the doctors' station. "For the excellent nurses and doctors," she said, her voice floating with song, eyes meeting ours, hands gaily waving, her unabashed sincerity rounding out her beauty.

Mrs. Tomczak sometimes varied the routine by bringing a double chocolate cake or maybe it was triple chocolate. The cake, soft in the white bakery box with fudge spilling over the lid, long flecks of coconut clinging to the inside, and the perfect maraschino cherry spotted directly on the cake's center. We would wolf down the sweet sustenance and whisper muffled gratitude.

My medical team was on call for the Code-One when Bill suffered another heart attack. He was blue, grabbing his chest, his blood pressure unobtainable, the electrocardiogram revealing a ventricular pattern, fast, wide, and irregular. Intravenous procainamide to establish a normal rhythm, pressor medications to raise his blood pressure, chest compression to provide oxygen, we worked desperately to save him, employing all of our tricks, and for too long, way too long, but nothing worked.

Every death was remembered in medicine. There's a depot for these tragedies in the brain, smack in the middle somewhere, maybe stored in the amygdala or hippocampus. Bill, young, handsome, hearty, was close to us in life—his death stood out—he was an outlier; and nothing dwelled inside us to help a third-year medical resident buffer the fragility of life and grief was notoriously difficult to share.

Sitting at the nurses' station, we discussed alternate professions. Perhaps baggage handling at the airport, an eight-hour day, two fifteen-minute breaks, thirty minutes for lunch, something physical and exhausting and devoid of sorrow. That was when the service elevator released the grim-faced morgue attendant pushing his gurney, and the passenger elevator discharged the smiling and gift-bearing Mrs. Tomczak. Waving to us, making sure we spotted her arrival, Amy turned left down the hall toward Bill's room, walking her quick, noisy steps. Everyone went head down on the writing ledge, busily occupying themselves with parsing sentences or composing letters to Santa. When God absents himself, it's difficult for mortals to provide cover.

“Mrs. Tomczak, please don’t go in there,” I implored. The only brave heart with voice, I stood up, ready to stop her progress. Studying my face, she understood everything.

“Bill’s dead, isn’t he?” she asked, her right hand moving over her chest, as if offering her heart for her husband. Amy stood motionless and vulnerable in the spare hospital hallway, jostled by the candy stripers and medicine carts, and in a gesture two millennia old, she crossed herself.

I nodded, “*Bill’s dead,*” I said. It was difficult for me to find voice.

“Doctor,” she said, politely, formally even, beckoning to me with her free hand. “Please come with me, I want to see Bill.” Precisely placing the bakery box with today’s offerings on the chair outside Bill’s room, she looked at me and spoke without rancor or cynicism: “Doughnuts for the good doctors and nurses.” God was unfair and inept, not us.

“This will be the last time Bill and I kiss,” Amy said. The injustice began to sink in. Bill, the person she loved and cherished, lying flat in bed, still and cold, eyes closed, the hospital gown back in place and tied around the waist. She ignored the Code-One debris of empty syringes and remnants of the emergency kits haphazardly tossed—medicine vials, gauze, tape, sponges, and tears—the Hieronymous Bosch version of hell: dead body, decaying lilies facedown in their fluted vase, scattered pillows encased in tight clear plastic reflecting the dull yellow haze from the once-white walls.

“Amy, scream, throw yourself against the wall. Life’s unfair. Bill didn’t have a chance. He had another major heart attack.” My speech made little sense. Of course it was major and yes, Bill hadn’t had a chance, otherwise he’d still be here.

Made awkward by the disorder of death, Amy kissed her Bill and placed her hands on his for a long minute, her eyes shut, her lips silently moving with prayer.

“What do I need to do now? And what about our plans, the plans Bill and I made?”

“I’ll sign the death certificate and contact the funeral home. And your plans with Bill, those plans,” I said, and paused, because it was my heart skipping beats. “We plan for good things, but the bad just has a way of happening.”

Amy laughed, the soft, inward laugh of a victim trying to marshal her strength, knowing her life had irrevocably changed and I hadn't offered comfort.

"Thank you, Doctor. I do need some assistance. If you can, walk me to my car, don't let me faint or break down or some sissy thing like that. Maybe you have a handkerchief or something for these damn tears? I don't want to get your shirt wet." She hugged me hard, head down, one quiet sob, gaining strength from human contact.

The long walk to the visitors' parking lot happened fast, stepping aside for mothers cuddling newborns and parents shepherding giggling children with colorful balloons tied in knots to their wrists. There's life and there's sadness in this place—it's just the way it is and it never changes—the hospital is always the hospital.

"I'm okay," Amy said, keys out, ignition turned, car started, and her every movement precise and in slow motion. "Doctor, thanks for your kindness, let's meet again during happier times." Head down, hands white, too tight on the steering wheel, turning away from me, carefully positioning the lever down to Drive, she raised the driver's-side window and wove her way out from the parking lot into the street.

My tour of Bill's room was an excuse to regain composure after my visit to the dark side of life. Bill's open wallet stared at me. It had fallen next to the bedside table with his driver's license face-up. It was scary how much Bill and I looked alike, maybe more like my cousin Charles, but with a broader forehead and a receding hairline. I hadn't noticed it before. I took the wallet to the nursing office to be sent to Amy and pocketed the driver's license.

The obituary was in the next day's newspaper. So sterile, with all the "beloveds," the listing of family members, the death "sudden"—yes, it was sudden—but nowhere in the boxed epistle were the tears or the sadness. Where did it say, here was a good man who deserved more time on earth?

I telephoned Amy several days after the burial and offered my condolences. "Doctor, thanks for the wishes, and don't even think about saying no, because we must have lunch together. I need medical information for my children, and I need to know about Bill's last day on earth. I dwell on it. I can't help it. Bill's face, the one in our wedding picture, youthful, handsome Bill with the scraggly mustache he loved so, is becoming smaller and smaller in my dreams, like Alice's Cheshire Cat."

We met at a local breakfast and lunch diner. Peter, the middle-aged owner, a friendly and happy maître d', coordinator, cook and busboy was always glad to see me and my companions, who were raucous, or attractive, or both. Today it was Amy, quiet and good-looking, comfortable in a pale yellow dress with flower imprints, cinched to her narrow waist with a wide midnight-blue belt, the color matching her eyes.

A grill adjacent to a closet-sized kitchen, one cook, and a menu four pages long with a hundred items, ranging from crab cakes to souvlaki, the latter their specialty: a little grilled pork and colorful vegetables, all fresh and delicious. The restaurant was modest, indeed, but the salads always arrived cold and the rolls warm. I ordered souvlaki for the two of us.

We talked about Bill. The last minutes of Bill's life made gentler by time and choice. No pain, eyes closed, arms folded, and his spirit levitating and then ascending to higher places or wherever spirits find their way, silently mouthing "*I love you Amy.*"

It was bullshit, but good bullshit.

"Your children need to see their pediatrician, exercise regularly and eat a well-balanced diet." I provided the summation of everything I knew about the ways of a healthy heart, none of which had helped Bill. Truth was we often touted our ignorance as gospel.

Solace travels many pathways. Our phone conversations drifted away from Bill. Grief and bereavement and rebirth and lust chased each other around and around, like the hands on a clock as generous as Big Ben, offering hope and resolution. Life's emotions were scattering like light traveling through a glass prism.

"I need a hug and a kiss," Amy said.

"So do I," I replied.

❖ ❖ ❖

I met Amy at a hotel near the airport. She'd booked a room for us.

After late-afternoon beers and talk about the weather, doctor work and nothing else important, we walked through the lobby, edging past the businesspeople, already restless, waiting for early-morning meetings and speeches, pausing to admire Amy's beauty, and envious of my good fortune, their salacious stares difficult to suppress. The suits in the crowded elevator turned silent, barely making space for us, pushing us together, our hands folded into one another.

We made love. "Yes Doctor," she said over and over. Her beautiful face was buried into my chest, eyes as closed as her world had become. Then we napped; the grumble of the window air conditioner the only intrusion. When we awakened, our closeness changed pedestrian dreams to passion once again.

The surreal contrast between thoroughly satisfying sex, both physical and ethereal, clashed oddly with the aftermath verbiage spooling forth about movies, books, and her children. We munched on tuna melts, fries, and vegetable chili among the clatter of the hotel's overpriced eatery, while I doodled on the paper napkins, closing the circles and the circles within circles, nothing left undone. The waitress brought us carrot cake, their specialty, *gratis*, she said, winking at us both in turn, assuming we were honeymooners.

# EIGHTEEN

Howard and Sophie listened to my description of my workweek and the meeting with Sergeant Esposito while we drove to Jane's parents' home for a Saturday night celebration. Sophie and I were on our best behavior for events such as these. Howard fit in naturally.

Sophie's loose-fitting summer dress, light yellow, the color of the midday sun, spotted with faint blue outlines of summer flowers—daisies, purple irises, and peonies—showcased her beauty as much as her tight shifts. Her hair, brushed straight down was soft and bouncy, her subtle-colored lipstick—light red with just a touch of pink—was not to be touched by external forces until later and hopefully only by me.

"The laboratory test results confirmed that Betty's lupus had been active," I said. I couldn't let go, breaking the silence of the travel. "And her husband is a *mal hombre*," I said, my high school Spanish right on the mark. Howard and Sophie retaliated in unison—"Stop with work details on an evening designed to be free from worries. Betty resides in a better place. Lupus is a bad disease, and you've already contacted the police about her husband."

"Ted, you did all you could for Betty Schmidt," Sophie said. "You're a good doctor, but you can't be everywhere. You and Dr. Raul checked on her, and she was improving. What more could you have done? We work with ill people and bad things happen all the time. You know that."

"But a private-duty nurse, or her transfer to the ICU, or me kicking Tim out, and the Schmidt children would have a mother and I could be at peace," I whined.

But screw those problems for now—we opened the bottle of gift wine. Jane's parents' elegant wine cellar wouldn't improve with our effervescent Portuguese rosé housed in its brown-colored crock. No opener needed, the polite *pop* predictably followed the unwinding of the coiled wire fastener keeping the mushroom cork in place. We finished off the sweet-tasting, fizzy liquid accompanied by Elvis Presley and Bill Haley medleys, and my thoughts about hospital work and Betty faded away.

The party, a valet-parking event, celebrated a promotion for Tom, one of Jane's siblings. The eldest son, now a full partner in a downtown law firm, was a good guy, smart, deserving of success and earning enough money to buy two or three internists. Howard and I took him and his buddy in basketball at their backyard court for the price of a good dinner. It wasn't close. Still we obsessively kept track of the score and argued about fouls until the end. We also partied together at Maddie's. Tom could be trusted to watch your back.

There was always a long and sinuous greeting line at Jane's house. It's an opportunity to greet eloquent and handsome people named Jinx or Binky or Bickers. You wanted to say those names over and over to yourself just for their resonance. The unfairness of it all, and it was so upfront, because not only were these guests rich, thin, and handsome, but they were bedecked in slinky and crisp stylish apparel—and I wasn't.

Tom and I laughed, pumped fists, and finally gave in and hugged. He wished to set a precedent for embracing Sophie, who was standing next in line.

We toured the palatial house. Tastefully decorated, extravagant rooms, and for this occasion, music everywhere, including a dance band in the parlor. Sophie estimated the wealth of the guests, whispering into my ear: "He's a partner—he's old money, possibly even *Mayflower* old," she said, her excitement ratcheting up for every million dollars. Her flirtatious banter and striking appearance entranced everyone, and she became the center of all the assemblages beckoning her.

"Ted, I'll dance with you later," she said, pushing me in the other direction. Sophie needed to organize her quest to meet the eligible men, single or otherwise, downplaying her statuesque loveliness with: "Oh shucks, I'm just a nurse," drawled down home-style, invoking libidinous fantasies of being tucked in, bussed, and massaged by Nurse Sophie. The recipients of her salutations reliving their cherished childhood memories of doctor and nurse games played out in the bedroom closet with cousins or neighbor kids, their parents away or busy sampling the dry sherry in the sunroom.

Howard and I raided the kitchen for beer. Wine was offered by a fleet of servants stationed in each room, but wine was for old people. Jane's father stocked the refrigerator with a Colorado beer called Coors just for the two of us—smooth, so very smooth. I carried a bottle in each hand.

Jane led me around and introduced me to her family for the tenth time; they were polite people with freely offered, expensive-looking smiles, remembering me, of course, and asking about the doctor business and my health.

Finally taking refuge in the library, I sat down next to a harp player with LYDIA printed on her nametag in large script, the badge attached to a pearl necklace snugly surrounding a long and graceful neck. Her black wool sweater was pulled down tight over the top of an inviting navy-blue, corduroy skirt stretched taut over her thighs, as her legs spread to accommodate the full-sized harp.

Harp playing wasn't just pulling strings and fluttering your hands while transposing Mozart. The utmost coordination was required between the foot pedal shortening the strings and raising the pitch, while both hands plucked the vertical strings, all forty-seven of them. Difficult, yes, very difficult, not too many men play one—okay, there were a few. But what guy in his right mind would carry a ninety-pound instrument around that needed constant tuning?

"Would you consider playing a duet with an accordionist and make me happy?" I asked her. "I grew up on music. Like you, it's in my soul," I said, my fingers moving vertically, mimicking the basic accordion scales.

❖ ❖ ❖

My mother had music in her blood. Our Victrola was stacked with every song recorded in Poland and America, and the music was accompanied by her cheerful soprano hum as she dashed between household chores. While my neighborhood friends were struggling with extracting sounds from the violin or piano, she signed a lifetime contract with an itinerant accordion teacher who came knocking at our door one morning.

Polite, low-keyed, and thrilled to find a Polish-speaking family in the neighborhood, he charmed Mother with just the right words: "The rental, conveniently paid weekly, is less than the investment in a piano, and the accordion is much less fragile than a violin." His hands snapped a pretend fiddle in half. "And the expensive violin strings need constant replacement. Why, just tuning the thing takes fifteen minutes and nobody actually gets it right. And a piano! Why those monstrosities take up half the space of your front room. Believe you me, Mrs. S, Chopin, the great one himself, would've played the accordion if his mother had been as smart and as attractive as you."

Mr. Tivorski proved to be an accomplished musician and teacher, and I was a receptive student. The accordion fit my busy personality, and the lessons kept me out of trouble. The tutelage only ended when I informed Mr. Tivorski—and it was said without rancor—that if I ever felt his hard wankel on my behind again, I'd throw him out the window. No notice, he just stopped coming after five years of lessons.

❖ ❖ ❖

A hint of a smile and Lydia, head down, her short dark hair bouncing skyward and returning without a strand out of place, plucked a popular song of the forties, a Rodgers and Hart composition from *Pal Joey*. The grandeur of her music was complemented by my singing.

*If you asked me, I could write a book*
*about the way you walk and whisper and look.*

My palms were held upward like I was reading a book, my eyes peeking at her from just above the faux pages.

Lydia, my Balthus seductress, was blessed with musical sweetness.

"Would you like a beer?" I asked after the duet, offering Lydia one of the two Coors I had orphaned on a table. "And when we walk in the rose garden, we'll talk about the harp. You'll be fascinated to know that paintings of them were found in Egyptian tombs thousands of years old. But, of course, no one as lovely as you was playing them."

No response to my scintillating patter! Lydia didn't appear to be an Abbott and Costello cinema aficionado, but who knows? Maybe I was the invisible man to her.

"Maybe English isn't your primary language and okay maybe they were lyres painted on the walls of the tombs and not exactly harps," I said, my alternate explanation for the snub.

"We'll travel wherever your heart desires, along, with our Berlitz teacher, and we'll book a separate room for your harp and maybe we'll dance a little."

Finally her mouth opened, the words reverberating from her lovely mouth as she carefully enunciated in proper English and without rancor—"Here I am stuck playing popular shit in this library room fifty miles out from the city with a goofus claiming to be a musician, who maybe knows about an undiscovered one-of-a-kind Bach or Mozart duet for accordion and harp. Oh my! Just my good fortune, a newly found harp and accordion manuscript! Listen to me carefully Mr. Nuisance, and read my lips: *Get lost.*" Her eyes finally met mine.

I've befriended a lot of women out of kindness in my lifetime, sometimes simply to boost their ego, and you'd think Lydia could've returned the favor. Even a full smile, or a laugh, just about anything would have been a victory. Heartbroken, I managed a thumbs-up, and since I usually follow instructions, moved on.

Sophie needed rescuing. With an insistent nod of her head, she gestured for help, while at the same time smiling and talking to a guest who was just a tad taller than her chest, which I'm sure was part of his fascination for my nurse.

"Ted, meet Phil. Talk business with him while I powder my nose."

"Wait Sophie," I said, "I'll go with you."

I didn't want to be stuck with Sophie's castoffs, and I grabbed her wrist.

"So Doc," said Phil, grabbing my arm in turn, shifting his focus to me, our trinity in place for better or for worse. "I'm from Bailey, Griddle and Brown, the investment bankers. Can you tell me what you think the trends are going to be in medicine for the next, oh, five to ten years?"

Assertive Phil, short and stocky, overdressed for this casual affair with a snug-fitting, expensive dark suit, the jacket's lower button on the verge of surrendering to his paunch, and a tie with stripes too bold. He insisted on answers to his business queries and likely acted on them.

"Trends, five or ten years?" I repeated politely and humbly. "Phil, I'm a medical resident. I do the scut work, start intravenous lines, do physical examinations, write laxative orders, check stools for blood, order the nighttime sedatives, inscribe notes to miss work or skip child support payments that kind of stuff. I don't know anything about trends." I graced him with my sincere smile and kept Sophie close, our fingers fighting for leverage.

Howard and Jane joined us. So, of course the inevitable happened.

"There is one thing, but it's still under wraps, Phil, and you'll need to promise not to make it public."

Phil happily nodded in the affirmative. It was as if we were offering Sophie to him for an evening of enchantment.

"It's new and exciting and will be a boon for many people, and perhaps even to you," I said.

"Hit me with it." Phil took the bait.

Phil was receiving hair transplants to fill in his expanding frontal bald spot. His dermatologist extracted plugs of hair from the sides of his head and inserted them in the front. A row of them were lined up, scraggly clumps of unhappy, misplaced follicles crowding his scalp.

"It's a new cosmetic procedure," I told him, gently fondling his balding pate, as if providing benediction.

"You procure hair plugs from clandestine, but fertile areas, in previously unused donor sites. In medicine, it's called a win-win situation."

Phil reveled in the analogy, nodding his head like a lost pup greeting a friendly face.

Jane chimed in, "How about the chest or back? They're wonderful sources of thick, manly hair."

Even mainline WASPs manage to join in the fun at their parties.

"Jane, dearest, the sexiest part of a guy is his back and chest hair. The woollier, the better. Now, a guy isn't going to give that up, is he? Am I right Phil?"

Phil nodded, yes, his excitement reaching a feverish pitch, what with new business opportunities on the horizon and Sophie still hanging around and her smile as beguiling as ever.

"I suspect you're a Jeff Chandler lookalike with your shirt off," I pointed to Phil. "Thick curly, macho stuff sprouting like ragweed—well we definitely don't want to take hair follicles from there."

Sophie, more disgusted than usual, probably did wish to move on and not miss attracting some of the prizes waltzing around the room. Maybe she would change into her nurse outfit and broadcast a need for a ride to work before stepping aside to avoid the stampede.

"If the source of the hair is down where I think it is, don't even mention it in mixed company," Sophie said.

"I'm flabbergasted with that suggestion," I said, my eyes shooting skyward before turning to Howard.

"Howard, is it okay to tell Phil and the ladies the source of the hair?"

"Of course, Dr. Ted, anything for our new buddy Phil." Howard, as helpful as always, placed his arm around Phil's shoulder.

"We harvest it from a hidden area. It has deeply colored, quality follicles with splendid growth potential. Everyone will be requesting it, even guys who are barely thinning on top. We'll open walk in clinics just for the procedure—first come, first serve and cash up-front. We're talking about nasal hair, of course," I declared, our throwaway punch line, and Howard and I were ready to move on.

Sophie took my hand and ordered, "Let's dance." Jane and Howard joined us. We thanked Phil for the sparkling conversation and left him in deep thought.

Dancing is serious business. Howard and I attribute our success in attracting women to our dancing skills, Lydia the harpist a notable exception. In the scientific world, she would be labeled an "outlier."

Strange, isn't it, when you think about it? You can be the ultimate goof, but if your feet move graciously when the music starts, life holds magnificent rewards. Every society visited by history—primitive, established, rich, poor, randomly chosen, whatever criteria you want to use, you'll find one constant, and that's a love of dancing.

"What do we do when we want to please the ladies after an afternoon of lovemaking?" I would ask Howard.

"Please them! I know exactly what to do to please them," he would shout.

"We dance," we'd sing out loud, our hands jiving.

"Please dance with me," the ladies beg. Their first "please" in two years and it's not about orgasms, bank accounts, jewelry, or anniversaries. "It's 'please dance with me,'" and they melt in our arms.

But you have to be dragged to the dance floor, be "put out" by the request. This is true. "Just one dance and it has to be a slow one," you begrudgingly whisper. Then you take charge and lead the way, slowly at first, and as the music pounds faster and faster, as it always happens, the band quickening the tempo, you spin your partner to the point of vertigo. Visions of Rudolf Nureyev sweeping them to ecstasy crowd their fantasies.

"Maybe one more dance," you say. "But then let's stroll outside and catch our breath." That's the moment when you go all-out. Twirls, hands up, spins, flashing feet, and you thank her for her skills, exuding sincerity, offering a quick and chaste hug, anticipating a lot more later.

And it works.

Sophie was content with the dancing, but then we bumped into Estelle and Fineglass, lost in their private reverie, staring blissfully at one another. That was unacceptable.

"Sophie, there's medical business that I need to talk to Dr. Estelle about," I said and edged her toward Howard. "Keep Sophie happy for a moment," I asked. Howard and I were able to exchange favors like that without a word of explanation. But just then, Phil butted in, assuaging my guilt for deserting my nurse. Spoken politely, but insistently, he said, "Let me have the honor of dancing with the loveliest lady on the North Shore. Thank you, Doctor," and swept my luckless beauty away.

"Estelle, Fineglass, sorry to interrupt," I said, moving over a few steps, rudely stopping them in mid step.

"Fineglass, I want to apologize about the fracas the other day. I was under a lot of stress, what with the death of my patient, then my grandmother passing away so suddenly, and me so unexpectedly running out of my chocolate laxative tablets. I left the lifesaving stuff out in the sun and they melted into a single concretion. All those setbacks happening on the same day, can you believe my misfortune? So please excuse me and pardon me once more, while I dance with Estelle. Medical business, you wouldn't understand."

Zero for two, another Lydia the harpist stare. Estelle was not happy with my sophisticated and slick dancing maneuvers.

"Estelle, I don't know how to say this graciously, but that night when we were together, you might vaguely remember the occasion, for me the event has taken over my life. I ruminate about the glory of that star struck occasion. It's a lot different for guys," I said. "And it's difficult for me to explain what I can't explain, but gosh, those damn things live forever. Such a mystery, something so brief and yet so enduring, as if snowflakes had touched our lips and spelled *infatuation*, one letter at a time. Yes—one letter at a time—*i, n, f*—well you get the point, and believe me, I can do better. Tell yourself minutes rather than seconds better. Next time, maybe we can even take our clothes off. Plus, what do you see in Fineglass?"

"You're cute Ted," Estelle responded. "Maybe if you'd convert, grow up, develop a personality and get rich, you'd be passable. Also, a little higher and harder would be nice, but thanks for being so persistent. And Ted, some words of wisdom from Kafka. You know, Franz Kafka. 'There's an infinite amount of hope in the Universe, but not for you.'" A soft cheek-kiss and Estelle departed in the middle of a slow and romantic two-step.

Jane's mother, beatific smile on her Katharine Hepburn face, tinkling a goblet with a golden spoon, asked everyone to gather in the parlor for the entertainment, the room large enough to accommodate Texas.

She congratulated Tom on his promotion, her clapping hands inviting widespread applause, proud of her eldest, and he was a conspicuously handsome son, followed by the announcement that Howard, her future son, would play a song or two. Howard was always asked to entertain.

Scarlatti's "Sonata in A," the music intertwining on itself like a Bach fugue followed by Mozart's "Rondo Alla Turca," were always crowd-pleasers. Howard knew his audience. Head down while playing—this could have been a Carnegie Hall recital. Add a candelabra and longer teeth, and Howard would be the medical profession's Liberace.

Thanking his audience, Howard announced a special treat. Jane, Sophie, and Ted would join him in a medley for Tom and Jane's parents and the lovely partygoers. The four of us singing "Love Me Tender" usually sung by Elvis Presley and "Chances Are," a 1957 hit by Johnny Mathis: *Chances are you think that I'm in love with you.*

We were good. Sophie wouldn't let go of my hand, forgiving me for the dance floor desertion.

Howard was staying overnight at Jane's, separate rooms of course, and Sophie and I drove Howard's car back to my apartment. Howard would come to work on Monday with Jane.

Jane's mother hugged us as we left, thanking us for the entertainment, thanking us for being in their lives.

"Ted, how is Dr. Rhimes?" she asked. "You do remember me telling you, he's a good friend of the family. When you see him, please give him my best."

# NINETEEN

How was Dr. Rhimes? The chief was fine. It was me who remained in his doghouse. The fiasco had occurred back in 1958, when I was still a first-year medical resident. I had convinced my senior resident, Jack Springerman, an IntMed 3, to let me discuss the patient with an unusual illness.

The chief conducted walking rounds two afternoons a week, along with the medical residents, discussing patients of interest. We inhaled the knowledge quicker than the supersized wet vacs sold at Montgomery Ward, while we marched from patient to patient. The chief matched wits with us, and we diligently prepared for these sessions, striving to impress him with our skills.

Quietly listening to our presentation, the chief would stand at the bedside, taking in everything—our words, the patient's appearance, the laboratory tests—and then he would perform his methodical examination. Head down in concentration, he isolated himself from the hospital chaos, immersing himself in the business at hand, and he missed nothing.

Pausing a few seconds to play with his pipe, he would tap the bowl on his palm several times and explain the thought processes allowing him to arrive at the diagnosis. The über teacher, the chief was medicine's aurora borealis, enlightening us, probing us, and clearing away our fuzzy thinking. Finally he would ask our plans for the patient to be sure we were on the right track.

I envisioned him carefully examining our Mr. Miller. Puzzled at first, with a slight frown, there might even be a trace of uncertainty, until his supercharged neurons integrated the information. And then a smile would light his face, and he'd turn toward me, acknowledging my challenge with a glance, eye contact established before he would announce: "Problem solved."

Two sophisticated physicians, he and I. Oh, the points I would garner! After asking the other residents and students to examine the patient, he'd walk over and place his arm around my shoulder, offering congratulations for the fascinating and educational afternoon.

It turned out, however, that the chief was never the best heart examiner. Throwing his hands up in exasperation after performing the physical examination, he smiled briefly at Mr. Miller. An insincere smile. And it wasn't a promising turn of events when he turned toward me, light absent from his demeanor, and asked: "So, what's going on here?"

Mr. Miller was in the hospital septic with a sinus infection and pneumonia, but recovering well with intravenous antibiotics. Anxious to please the doctors surrounding his bed, he told his story of repeated infections and the wonderful surprise they had in store for them when he disclosed his secret.

I had performed the initial history and physical examination when Mr. Miller was admitted to the hospital. He regaled me with his life story, but he didn't mention the abnormalities he was born with, but by then, the on-call radiologist had paged me and informed me that either the technician screwed up the right/left marker on the chest X-ray, or Mr. Miller had dextrocardia, or even *situs inversus*, with the stomach bubble on the right side, not on the left where it belonged.

*Bang* and *crash* circled my cerebrum, now I knew why the physical examination confused me with the heart sounds being more prominent on the right side of his chest. Mr. Miller's heart was on the wrong side!

Kartagener's syndrome was a rare disorder with the heart and often all the internal organs inverted. There were frequent sinus and lung infections. The chief didn't pick it up. He didn't even listen over the right side of the chest. He didn't appreciate the left-sided liver or the right-sided descending colon. Trouble wafted around us that was more pervasive than the stink from the nearby Union Stockyards.

Mr. Miller didn't help the situation, opening his big mouth in spite of my admonishment to remain silent during the entire session under penalty of being prescribed a low-salt, no fat, limited fluids, low-calorie diet with extra-steamed broccoli, and anything else I could think of to make his life miserable.

"Hey, Doc," Mr. Miller said to me, *sotto voce*, "the old guy didn't get the diagnosis, did he?"

Now turning toward the chief, finger pointed his way, he crowed, "Hey, Mr. Big Shot Doctor, you screwed up, didn't you? Go ahead and admit it." His smirk was not at all endearing. "My heart's not where you placed your stethoscope thingy." Then he pointed to the right side of his chest and shouted gleefully. "Heart here!" He laughed, fist emphatically hitting his right chest. "My heart's here!"

I sidled in front of Mr. Miller, masking his jeering and whispering to him that his lack of cooperation was going to cost him dearly.

The chest X-ray demonstrating the right-sided heart stirred no huzzahs from the chief. No "good work, job well done smiles" extended to me or to my resident. I left out the "of course" when I discussed the diagnosis and focused on mundane issues such as bowel habits and oral hygiene.

I was never forgiven for stumping our blessed chief.

"Shithead" was Jack Springerman's moniker for me for the remainder of the month. Jack and I have not maintained a friendship.

# PART THREE

# ONE

## *Winter 1961*

On crutches and recovering from the now-infamous baseball-bat beating, I looked at mug shots at the Third Police District. Wounds caused no comment in this place. The station was weekday busy, desks abutting, enough telephones for a bookie joint and all being used. Lord knows what was being talked about, but it must have been business because the rumble of whispers and shouts included a plethora of the "f" word.

All of the desks were occupied and cigarette smoke spiraled in every direction. By and large, these were regular-appearing people. Facial stubble, jangling handcuffs, grunts, lip edges pointing downward—and those were the *good* guys, the ones not being given the third degree. Maybe the denizens here were bigger than most, and regular people generally didn't have revolvers strapped to them.

I found it difficult not to stare at the weapons since my childhood had been spent fantasizing about six-shooters and bad guys hitting the dust after a barrage of hot lead. Every curved piece of wood, every plastic utensil—knives, forks, you name it—everything fondled in childhood was loaded with bullets and aimed at cattle rustlers and enemy combatants foolishly strolling through the neighborhood.

Big Guy and my baseball bat swinging friend weren't in the mug shots. Grammar school classmates were scattered here and there in the loose leaf binder of bad actors, but not the two guys who'd caught my attention so professionally and left my face so pristine, my good fortune, of course.

The sergeant had visited Tim at his office, making sure the squad car that hadn't been washed in a year blocked the entrance, passenger-side tires on the curb. But that infringement of Tim's space likely enhanced his reputation. Tim was told that harassment of doctors would end with punishment that was not necessarily court-dictated. I didn't point out to the sergeant the ineffectiveness of the warning.

George said to stay away from Tim. They would continue to watch him. And the sergeant was presenting the information I provided about Betty to the assistant district attorney.

"But I think it's hopeless for now, Doc. Maybe we'll catch Tim in another mistake. You know Maria Amaroso left the country. It's my thinking that Tim's goons played a house call on her. She left for the Philippines a few days ago and she didn't tell me a thing. *Nada*! She had my card."

❖ ❖ ❖

My mother and stepfather stayed around to play the indulgent parents while I recovered from my injuries. Harry, now retired from Pharmacy, helped me with my transportation and picking up the books and medical records that kept my mind occupied. The hospital had retracted their offer of travel assistance, not wanting to establish a precedent for being helpful.

The neighbors had formed a citizen watch group. Mrs. Linderman, my seventy-six year-old next-door friend, and I shared the second-floor landing. One sixty-watt bulb dangled unadorned between us that needed changing every other week, a duty that I graciously performed, while standing on my rickety folding chair. In return, she promised to look after me.

"Lots of excitement you're having," she commented on the extent of my recent beating. "Who would have thought a podiatrist could have so much adventure? It's better than shaving corns."

"I'm studying to be an internist, not a podiatrist," I informed Mrs. Linderman, once again cognizant that information might dampen our relationship. Disappointment registered on her face, as she wrestled with accepting my lesser status. Finally, she found a compromise and asked me, as an amateur of course, to take a gander at her malformed piggies.

The reward for my enthusiastic appreciation of her corn-laden toes was sincerely offered. "Mr. Internist-in-Training, if you ever need help with the bad guys, let me know. We'll have a secret signal, maybe like you phoning me or knocking at my door and asking if I'm wearing my skimpy, silk pajamas, the shiny pink ones that open in front with one pull of the lace bow, or some other neat password and I'll hustle over with my Smith & Wesson. It's a .38 special, semiautomatic limited-edition beauty with a pearl handle and an adjustable trigger stop that shoots death.

"It's heavy, so I have to use two hands," she continued. No old-age tremors were present when she demonstrated her grip. "You know what semiautomatic means, don't you? A foot doctor would know that."

I didn't know what semiautomatic meant, and I didn't relish this discussion that was so far out of my league. Mrs. Linderman was beginning to remind me of Mrs. Gail or Mrs. B. Maybe she was their aunt.

"Semiautomatic means that the gun is cocked and ready to go after each firing," she explained. "It's great when there's two or more of them. 'Come and take my food stamps and my *bubbie's* sterling-silver candlesticks, will you, you motherfuckers, *bam, bam*, and they're blown away, first one, then the other. They're history." Mrs. Linderman jiggled her torso with each "*bam*."

"Just telephone or yell for me." She poked me in the ribs, then turned her walker around and hobbled away.

❖ ❖ ❖

Mother and Harry hosted a dinner party. Mother would cook like the old days, accompanied by copious amounts of red wine. Later, and after only a minimal amount of urging, out would come my accordion, joined by singing, clapping hands and shots of Sobieski vodka. Mother would be in second heaven. Her only complaint centered on my lack of a formal table covering and silverware. Clean plastic forks were used and serviceable, but Elmer Fudd cartoon napkins and matching tablecloth—the napkins precisely folded in triangles and artfully displaying the entire "*Shhhhh, be vewwwy vewwwy quiet*" trademark with Elmer, rifle in hand, quietly sneaking up on that rabbit acting badly—were not appropriately formal for this occasion.

"Tadeusz," she said with a Polish drawl she engaged on demand. "You can invite a girl if you wish." Mother was impressed that I even had friends to ask over, and she decided to press her luck.

But which girl? Amy had family business, and how would Mother receive Amy, several years my senior and a recent widow with two children? Estelle was on call, plus her untimely engagement to Fineglass threw a monkey wrench into party plans. "*Higher and harder*," sung to the strains of the popular song, "The High and the Mighty," were sung to me at every opportunity.

"Sophie, dearest, it's Ted. How about coming over for dinner? No, you won't need to stop to pick up the carryout. No, it's not cold noodles with ketchup like last time. And those noodles were fresh, barely a week old, and it wasn't completely my fault about their color, okay, although you're right about one thing, I might have forgotten to refrigerate them. And Jane and Howard will be here and you know they have high standards." I paused for a second before delivering the coup de grâce: "And my mother and stepfather will be here."

Inviting your girl to meet your parents was so very high in the scheme of pleasing women that Sophie became speechless. I'll need to add it to my repertoire. It was more effective than displaying baby pictures or walking a taffy-colored cocker spaniel puppy. A rent-a-mother service would go over bigger than a Mormon family reunion.

Dinner was a success. Sophie kissed my mother and flirted with Harry. I hadn't seen him blush before, while he followed her from kitchen to dining room and back, talking nonstop about music, current events, movies, more conversation than I had had with either of them for years.

Sophie's hair, combed straight back, tight, exposed her flawless skin and her black wool skirt hung down to her knees, fetchingly bouncing north and south. A silky dark blue blouse complemented her azure eyes. She appeared the ingénue, and I loved her for it. Thoughts of Amy and Estelle faded fast.

I promised to please Sophie when the opportunity arose. Talk sweetly after lovemaking, participate in meaningful conversation, and then later prepare the scrambled eggs, just as she liked them, firm with the green peppers and onions sautéed first for several minutes and then served hot right after she showered and dressed for work.

Jane and Howard, naturally polite and good conversationalists, also charmed the folks. Howard gushed over the Côtes du Rhône rouge that Harry selected, able to talk the talk of an oenophile. The wine was too light for Polish dining, but guzzled by all without complaint. Mother prepared dinner, cooking everything from scratch, and at the same time managing to talk to us and laugh at the punch lines. She was the mother, and the kitchen belonged to her. "The food honors my late husband," she said, "and it pleases my son and Harry. What else could a mother want?"

"The *pierożki* are Tadeusz's favorite," said as Mother served the sauerkraut and cheese-filled dumplings that were foreign to me. Where was her thick, rich corned beef set next to the firm potatoes sprinkled with paprika that comprised the mainstay of our special occasions?

Her words were mixed with delightful idioms, asking me if I still breakfasted on "*cheery-oats*." Sentences caromed as fast as her purposeful steps, and her sensible shoes kept her flying between kitchen and dining room. Harry reveled in her peasant girl routine. And she never passed up an opportunity to stroke his face or hand.

Then came a sample of her specialty, hard-boiled eggs stuffed with ham. "Sticks to the ribs," she said, and Mother pinched Jane's cheek. She suggested weight gain for both of the ladies, although Mother carried no extra pounds. Mother had maintained her sturdy good looks with constant movement and youthful genes. With the omni loving graciousness of a doting mother and wife, she worked hard to please Harry and me.

I'm not sure when she'd last made this ultra-caloric dinner, but our health-conscious dining crowd couldn't get enough of it. It brought back my memories of a family Friday night or an Easter Day treat when our guests were greeted at the door with pickled herring chopped with apple, celery, and dill pickle mixed with sour cream, vinegar, and homemade mayonnaise, spread thickly on bits of rye bread. A conversation stopper, it caused a sudden intake of breath, the taste buds traveling ecstatic over the multitude of delights, signaling the brain to stop and enjoy. I used the quiet the delicacies produced to size up the visitors.

Our dinner was filled with laughter, family on an overdue holiday; we were a contented bunch, enjoying the coffee and honey cake, while I narrated the poem my father had treasured:

### Happiness

I asked the professors who teach the meaning of life
to tell me what is happiness.
And I went to famous executives who boss the work of
thousands of men.
They all shook their heads and gave me a smile
as though I was trying to fool them.
And then one Sunday afternoon I wandered out along
the DesPlaines River
And I saw a crowd of Polanders under the trees with
their women and children and a keg of beer and an accordion.

Years after my father's death, in my introductory poetry appreciation class, which the apathetic Mr. Kennedy taught to an abundance of laggards, Mr. Kennedy laughed for the first time, perhaps for the first time in a decade, and corrected my Carl Sandburg.

"Mr. Ted, get the original poem out. I think the poet wrote, 'Hungarians,' not 'Polanders.' Correct me if I'm wrong, but it's a great poem in any case."

He was right on both accounts.

Howard and Harry talked business, stocks, real estate, wine, art investments. And Sophie and Jane talked to Mother like old friends or sisters, while I busily fiddled with my decrepit television set, trying to find the football scores.

There were sparks when Sophie and I touched, as she helped me with my crutches and with sliding my chair in and out. Nurse and patient. And later we took advantage of the romantic aura with gentle love and then not-so-gentle love, working off the huge meal and ignoring my stiff leg and tender chest. I kept my promise and tended to Sophie's needs, even incorporating Estelle's suggestions about location and intensity. We talked softly, described our pleasures, as my hands sculpted her body, and there were no distractions—our beepers placed on off mode and the telephone muffled. The world would be a happier and kinder place if everyone could make love to Sophie.

# TWO

Reading X-rays with the wizards sitting around the radiology department, I gleaned as much about the machinations of the stock market and investing strategies as I did about detecting hilar adenopathy and pneumothoraces. Time was proving kind, my wounds healing, my circadian rhythm normalizing, my face and cheeks beginning to fill out, and my color returning.

I arranged an interview with Dr. Mollman, the head of Hematology at the university for a fellowship position. Mrs. Gail assured me that, for better or worse, the chief would call ahead and speak to him. Herb Rhoban approved of my plans, volunteered to also telephone Dr. Mollman, and encouraged me to return and work with him after I completed laboratory training. It was difficult to find tennis player patsies.

University Hospital was a geographic maze, demonstrating facets of the chaos theory propagated down the street at the physics department. Their information signs were devised by Catskill-prepped comedians: Elevator N intersected Hallway G and Outpatient Elevator B; only the parking garage was less user-friendly. When I became hospital chief, institutional improvements would be high up on the agenda.

Dr. Mollman was pronounced "*moll-man*," as in *gun-moll*, not "*mole-man*," I was emphatically instructed. Imposing and pompous, and he had earned it, the discoverer of the role of structural chromosomal abnormalities underlying certain forms of leukemia—and he was also blessed with prematurely gray hair, a tall, slim body habitus and a regal carriage.

"You'll have to spend one year working in the laboratory before joining the clinical rotations because you're applying so late," he told me.

"Dr. Mollman,"—I pronounced his name crisply and accurately—"that's great. I *want* to spend a year in the lab. That's not punishment. I want to learn laboratory methods and the scientific process. But please, I don't want to be someone's tool and just spend time preparing solutions and following a stale recipe. Let me finish the year of research with some hope that I may someday become independent in the laboratory, and become famous, of course."

Dr. Mollman, his expression fixed and bland, wasn't used to supplicants making demands. On the other hand, that was what every research leader wanted to hear, an outspoken candidate who desired to work hard. "Pushy" was good in research circles. I smiled at him as an associate, and he returned my smile, relaxing, facial muscles softening and he asked me my interests.

"Understanding why we develop antibodies directed against platelets and what prompts their formation," I answered. Immobilization and confinement after the beating had provided me with time to organize my thoughts. "What sites are the antibodies attaching to? Why do they destroy some platelets and not others? Why do some lupus patients have a propensity to clot rather than bleed even when their platelets are decreased?" My questions were merging together like the bulls crowding the narrow passageways of Pamplona during their summer festival.

Dr. Mollman reminded me of the chief because he stopped and thought for a moment before answering. Maybe successful people usually think before speaking. Then he explained the vagaries of antibody production, and the role of lymphocytes that matured into plasma cells, ultimately synthesizing the antibodies I was interested in—it being an area of particular interest to Dr. John Brennan, one of his up-and-coming young researchers. "I'll have you meet him this afternoon and you'll tour his laboratory." And we shook hands like contemporaries rather than professor and laboratory fodder.

Several of the hematology fellows took me to lunch. The doctors at the university had their own restaurant, no cafeteria lines, no Mrs. B in your face—the duality of aggravation and resentment these people were missing could fill a library and leave a permanent void in their maturation—*remember* I wished to tell them, *without a hurt, the heart is hollow.*

Dr. Brennan reminded me that laboratory research was exciting, but physically exhausting. Weekends and night hours were usual. After my three years of medical residency burdened with Mrs. Gail's scheduling, hard work and long hours would never be a threat.

I pushed the envelope and asked for clinical time, perhaps a half-day clinic a week and participation in inpatient rounds. "I'm a terrific clinician," I told Dr. Brennan and it wasn't completely untrue. I didn't inform him that I also created controversy wherever I went.

Dr. Brennan used our meeting as an opportunity to describe his area of expertise. His research with antibody production from cell cultures would help me understand laboratory methods. I was a bonus for him and he made me feel wanted. The Section of Hematology would pay my salary while I worked in his laboratory, and my ideas meshed with his longtime goals.

This bench would be mine, he pointed out, and here was Sarah, a research associate from Argentina and an excellent selling point for joining Dr. Brennan. Sarah welcomed me to the lab with a firm handshake.

"Could we meet for coffee so I can better understand your research?" I asked her and flashed my million-dollar smile. It must have registered as nickels and dimes because she responded, "You're normal, aren't you, Ted, and if so, would you please donate blood? We always need controls."

"That's the nicest question anyone's asked me in years," I said. "Normal, well I'm indeed normal, I guess, as normal as any average twelve-year old."

"Sit here, extend your arm, we'll use you anyway," she replied, a wisp of a smile, as her soft hands placed a rubber tourniquet tight around my biceps for the venipuncture. My arm rested on her leg as she stroked the median cubital space, encouraging the veins to show themselves. The needle stick was unfelt as I memorized her precise face surrounded by dark brown hair, eyes almost black, sloe-eyed, exotic—apparently descendants of the Mongol hordes had representatives even in South America. Her confident smile resided on top of a compact figure ensconced in a loose white laboratory coat fallen open to reveal trim breasts and a light brown wool dress tight around the waist and thighs.

"Would you also desire my heart or liver?" I asked.

She laughed and said, "Neither, but maybe I'll have time for coffee. Come back after I spin the blood down, I really just want the plasma. I'm measuring antibodies to nuclear antigens in patients with low platelet counts and hopefully you'll be a negative control."

"That sounds denigrating, a *negative control.* I'd rather be a positive influence on you." She pressed a plug of cotton firmly over the venipuncture site covering it with a strip of white adhesive tape, then playfully offering a strip to cover my loose mouth. Forget about spinning iron bars around a magnet or other high school physics experiments generating electricity, her touch was more productive.

Sarah met me near the elevator, no white laboratory coat, so I could enjoy the swaying of her stride. Eyeglasses accentuated the seriousness of our meeting, serially removing them and rotating the plastic temples in her sensuous mouth, while describing her research and the pleasure of working with Dr. Brennan. Her charm accelerated time, until we realized the session had to close. She guided me to the parking lot and with the swinging doors and ninety-degree turns, our hands and bodies lightly touched enough times to continue the flux of electrons. Her home phone number was provided with hesitancy.

"I have a boyfriend at home in Argentina, you know." She told me this with great seriousness, eyes seeking mine. "A boyfriend slash fiancé-type boyfriend. He's an outstanding scholar, prominent family, etc., just to let you know this up-front," as our hands found each other.

"He's a lucky guy," I responded. "I have a girlfriend, several of them actually, no commitments slash engagements. And I'm tall and funny," I continued.

"But I'm prettier. Actually much prettier," she said and squeezed my hand.

# THREE

An afternoon coffee break with Nurse Sophie provided a wonderful respite in our long day of patient service. A sudden quiet in the flow of hospital activity allowed us to replenish our souls as we mixed medical business with romantic murmurings. My hands and psyche felt much more caring after gently stroking her white nylon-clad legs folded under the cafeteria table.

Sophie had traveled a difficult road. Her parents had separated early and her growing-up time was spent with her father with the assistance of various aunts and family friends. Father, a fireman, worked erratic hours. Mother, when sober, a loving person, but drinking problems led to illnesses and hospitalizations. Sophie's visits to her mother at the county's chronic care facility in Oak Forest sparked her interest in nursing. She absorbed the benefits of TLC. Nursing the wild critters harmed by civilization, the crippled birds and the squirrels surviving encounters with Ford and Chevy station wagons, sparked the first step; then came the abandoned cats and dogs, and later the human beings.

Statuesque, with a Daisy Mae persona, she was perfect, and I've searched for flaws. Sophie stopped traffic. The unique problems posed by her beauty complicated the mixed signals of adolescence. Prohibited from dating until she was sixteen, with just a few minor mishaps along the way and those with older guys, too muscled for her to strike back, she survived the teenage years, completed her education, and began the better life that her mother had talked about during lucid moments.

Sophie won a scholarship to the best academic nursing school in the city and became a legend. A diligent, bright student during the week and a Playboy Bunny on weekends, she enthralled the newspaper public with her admixture of talents. But they were really the same, weren't they? Simply, providing comfort to people in need.

Courted by every VIP admitted to 3GM, even the wives would plead with the nursing supervisors to assign Sophie to their spouses. Recovery was infinitely quicker when lying straighter in bed, stoic, no whining, polite, hair combed neat—the post discharge withdrawal from her beauty could be dealt with later.

We saw each other daily, and in our own way, we were true to one another. The multitalented Mrs. B, noticing our entrance into the cafeteria announced our arrival: "No hand holding, no smooching, no touching in the dining area—not here"—stretching out the "*here*" with more pizzazz than the sidekicks on the late-night television shows.

"You won't guess whom I'm going to New York with this weekend," Sophie matter-of-factly told me.

"Sophie dearest, it's James Dean or Rock Hudson or both, if there's fairness in this world," I replied.

"It's Phil," she said calmly, as if she was giving a nursing report.

"Phil, as in Jane's party, the venture capitalist, that Phil?" I managed to ask.

I'm good at handling surprises, but Sophie could read me like a Las Vegas blackjack dealer.

"Don't give me that look," she said. "Life is so much easier for us girls. I told Phil at Tom's party that I liked Broadway music and *voilá* that's French by the way, we're off to see *The Sound of Music*."

"Sophie, after you hear the silly songs, and Phil primps his hair follicles, what are you two going to do? He's too big to stuff in the closet."

"Life is simple; there's a quid pro quo as they say in Norwegian. Tight silk panties, black or red, his choice, sit on his chin for a few minutes, and then its jewelry shopping, dinner, the musical, and home."

"Okay, I fully understand," I was nodding my head in agreement, fully appreciating the soundness of her plan.

# FOUR

Dr. Trillup arrived. The kidney doctor based at the university was famous for his insights into the pathogenesis of lupus. He had popularized the use of kidney biopsies to assess disease activity and dictate treatment. I was enamored with his dynamic and evidence-based approach to ill patients.

Dr. Trillup insisted we provide medical information in an orderly fashion. Crucial to meticulous patient care was the minutiae of management: the diet, the sodium load, urine output, precise weights, blood pressure control, and monitoring serum-albumin levels. There was a precise rhythm to his approach to the sick, and we acquired discipline when we interacted with him. We also were pleased that Dr. Trillup was based at the university and not at our hospital because he was a *schmuck*.

A lean, handsome man with thick dark hair combed straight down over his ears, a perfect midline part stolen from Prince Valiant, and a chiseled face, he was a walking advertisement for a successful physician. But, good looks and intelligence should have brought peace and decency. He was a bully.

Dr. Trillup needed someone to blame when things turned sour, as they often did in medicine, especially with patients burdened with chronic diseases such as lupus. A thrower, a skill usually reserved for prima donna surgeons, he tossed the chart or tray of food or bundle of sponges or whatever became handy with Torquemada intensity at residents or students who angered him by not meeting his expectations. And since his unhappiness could happen so quickly and unexpectedly, it remained best to stay out of his line of fire. My size and demeanor gave him second thoughts about attacking me, but my loose mouth made me eligible for verbal outbursts. I had elicited his unhappiness more than once. Possessed with a short memory, by the next day he had forgotten who had been his target.

Like many famous combatants, Dr. Trillup was accompanied by kind disciples astute enough to warn us when they sensed an eruption. This year, it was an old friend, Sandy Fong. Senior by one year to me, she was still a colleague and had been the only Asian American in her medical school class. Helpful, fun, smart, and generally capable of cajoling Dr. Trillup away from his random and spontaneous aggression, she also was perceptive enough to laugh at my attempts at humor.

And I learned from Dr. Trillup. One forgives childish behavior from smart people who are effective teachers. Like a professional golfer who demonstrated how to handle the short irons, Dr. Trillup taught us fundamentals that kept us ahead of the pack.

A special morning report, the chief attended, Wendy was featured with her two-by-two inch Kodachrome slides and carousel, and so was Sergeant Esposito, in plainclothes, no revolver in sight, presumably not anticipating a shootout and trying to be as unobtrusive as only a city policeman could be when attending a medical conference. Dr. Rosenthal sat in the back trying to appear small while fumbling for his calming medicine stored in his suit coat side pocket. Betty's death was not his doing.

Chuck, the chief resident, was nominally in charge, but I had preempted him and mailed my presentation to Sandy for forwarding to Dr. Trillup. I wanted Dr. Trillup to be prepared, or maybe *forewarned* was a better word choice. He was my hope for sorting out the events of that tragic night.

I took my time presenting Betty's history and hospital course, focusing on eye contact, voice modulation, and key points, describing Tim's behavior and the physical marks he had left on Betty. Howard interpreted the X-rays and electrocardiograms, and professionally so, because we had painstakingly reviewed the material the night before. Chuck, the chief resident, commented about the routine laboratory results. Test results assessing the activity of lupus needed more expert explanation, and Chuck graciously, as instructed, yielded to Dr. Trillup.

Dr. Wendle described the pathology findings. Assured and well-prepared and as imposing as Dr. Trillup, she selected autopsy slides revealing inflammation at multiple sites, the pericardium and myocardium, pleura, mesentery, and intestine. And she presented her version of the renal findings, although the kidney pathology slides also were reviewed by the pathologists at the university.

I queried Wendy: "If we biopsy a routine lupus patient who walks in off the street with mildly active disease, would your findings be different from those in Betty Schmidt?"

"I don't know the answer for sure, but thanks for asking," she said. "As you know, Ted, there really is no routine lupus patient." She smiled over her words, because we had argued about this question the day before. "There was considerable inflammation in this patient," she continued, "and in many areas that represented undertreated lupus. Coronary artery inflammation and atherosclerosis were present, and it was more than you would see in the general population, but probably not unusual for a lupus patient with active disease who was receiving prednisone medication."

Wendy paused before continuing, and this time the smile was for everyone. "That was a long answer and an incomplete response to Dr. Ted's question, but it's the best I can do. I believe it's the best anyone can do. Lupus is a complicated disease and the scales for measuring injury and inflammation are arbitrary. There were no signs in the autopsy that a physical struggle had taken place near the time of death," she added. "The bruises scattered over the patient's body were old. But asphyxiation, for instance, is often difficult to document." The latter was added for my benefit.

It was Dr. Trillup's turn. He politely acknowledged the chief, Wendy, and me, in that order, then began. The doctor pontificated best by walking around, hands deep in pockets, periodically and abruptly stopping and turning to face the attendees—a wonderful maneuver to keep his audience alert. I don't know if he owned a suit or sports coat or formal attire of any kind, because he was always bedecked in his crisp white doctor coat, rigid like medieval armor, but with starch not steel. Maybe it was part of his Prince Valiant motif. But Dr. Trillup would be sadly mistaken if he thought the city police would waive a speeding ticket because he was dressed as a doctor.

"This good young doctor,"—presumably meaning me—"had difficulties with the patient. It seemed that her symptoms suggested an abdominal crisis that, in the face of active lupus, could signal the presence of mesenteric vasculitis, which often requires surgical intervention." He emphasized his point by flicking his hair behind his ears using both hands. "Yet the autopsy didn't reveal severe vasculitis, and I'm sure that it was thoroughly searched for at this august institution."

More walking, hands deep in his pockets. "The kidney involvement was significant but treatable," he said, "and shouldn't have caused trouble at this time."

"I've seen many lupus patients," he continued, "and unfortunately, I've encountered sudden deaths." He grimaced and shrugged his shoulders, staring at his sidekicks as if they were the cause of the failures. "The deaths were most often due to myocardial infarctions, or pulmonary emboli," which echoed exactly what the chief told me months before. Dr. Trillup scratched his behind like a kid fending off pinworms, while explaining his great thoughts. "But this patient didn't have either, and I'm sure if they were present, the pathologist would have detected them. So perhaps there was an electrolyte abnormality or a sudden fatal arrhythmia, the latter a little surprising in the face of only modest myocardial inflammation."

The latter was identical to my interpretation, which no one had paid attention to.

He smiled. It was, as usual, a virtuoso performance—until Sandy Fong stood and asked: "Dr. Trillup, in light of such limited findings on the postmortem examination and the history of spousal abuse, should Dr. Ted have notified the police? Should homicide be considered a possibility? Dr. Wendle mentioned the search for asphyxiation, but then she seemed to vacillate about the findings."

*Thank you, Sandy. Thank you, thank you!*

Dr. Trillup loved being challenged by his favorite few. He thought for a moment, shrugged his shoulders once again, scratched his behind, and finally said, "I don't know the answers. Sometimes life ends abruptly in our ill patients, and often there's no good explanation. Part of our professional burden is trying to understand these events. It makes us want to continue our quest to become wiser." Then he gave Sandy a stern look before saying. "And then we move on."

The conference was over. Dr. Trillup thanked us for inviting him, and he and the chief left for their own tête a tête. I didn't know whether Dr. Trillup had an opinion about foul play or simply didn't want to go out on a limb, especially with George Esposito in the audience. Either way, I was crushed. My hope for justice for Betty's tribulations seemed lost.

I suppose I shouldn't have been surprised.

I hugged Sandy and Wendy, thanked Howard for "volunteering" to read the X-rays and Chuck, the chief resident, for his participation and for inviting Dr. Trillup. The sergeant was gone and I had no chance to hear his thoughts.

No one had offered a satisfactory explanation for Betty's death. Drs. Trillup and Wendy had skirted the issue. Nothing supernatural is occurring when we die. We don't just "pass away," or suddenly find that "Betty's gone," or "she's not here any longer." Death in a hospital shouldn't be a mystery, and my doctor experts were pussyfooting around for an explanation.

# FIVE

I traveled west on the Congress Expressway until it ended and then some. The landscape became rural, pumpkins piled higher than eyesight, autumn squash weighted between passageways, prairie and farmland beyond, oak trees shadowing the grass now yellow with the season. The pleasantness spread a patina of normality.

My Oldsmobile Rocket 88 was gray, sleek, with four doors, but not a family car unless the children sat snug and held on tight as I peeled away from the stop sign with a satisfying growl from dual exhausts. A gift from Harry and Mother, now ten years old, the Olds turned over every day with a welcome and sensuous roar. The glow of the whitewall tires after I scraped and buffed them would make them proud. The car was as reliable as the shadow of the frontal headache that greeted me on mornings when I was short of sleep. Today, the discomfort was magnified by awakenings throughout the night as I rehearsed my purchase. The car's heater, randomly on or off had no intermediate level and was going full blast for no discernible reason and was hot enough to fuel the throbbing that circled my head.

Al, of Big Al's Gun Shop, waited on me in person. Prosperous-appearing and gregarious, he resembled Jackie Gleason. Fat, sly, funny, and like the comedian, light on his feet. He'd move nimbly enough if I were an outlaw ordering him to dance while shooting bullets at his feet.

"I want an easy-to-use pistol and it should be compact, but then again, it should have stopping power." I gave my practiced recitation.

"These are the pistols I recommend," Big Al said, twirling a few, opening the chamber on others, stroking the handles on some, as we moved along his shelf of merchandise. "You've come to the right establishment for firearms when you're talking about velocity and impact, and when you want to add value. But in addition to making a profit, I want to please my customers." Big Al mixed his speech with the pantomimed draw of a phantom pistol from his empty waist holster and shooting the lights out.

"I've sold to the cream, you've heard of the Saint Valentine's Day Massacre, seven dead in less than a minute? Bugs Moran's gang enjoyed a permanent vacation thanks to Al Capone, my very own and special customer. Hey, just kidding about that." Big Al laughed, followed by a nudge to my shoulder. My caring salesperson was trying to interject humor and put me at ease. Or maybe he thought I was a movie producer casting a Western or gangster flick and needed a consultant.

The instruments of death excited my senses. The shiny dark metal handles rested snug in my palm and felt hefty and stone cold. "*Pow pow*," I aimed at the villains populating my childhood memories, replaying vengeful fantasies.

A sucker for sales pitches, I settled on a not-so-compact Smith & Wesson .45-caliber semiautomatic weapon. "The wide diameter of the bullet and its slower muzzle velocity reduces the possibility of passing through the target and injuring someone else," Big Al lectured. And I agreed. Pets, decorative art, and strangers wandering through the rooms needed protection.

"Big Al, if you'd apply your firearm wizardry to the establishment of world peace or explaining the White Sox collapse, the earth would be a better place," I told my new friend, making his day and prompting an energetic thumbs-up.

Big Al's corpulence required an expensive meal program, and I accepted his price without complaint. I was now a registered gun owner. The weapon, shiny, pristine, and wrapped up in gift paper, could pass for a cherished Christmas or birthday present for the kids or the little woman.

All of my lady friends had described their love of shopping in such reverent tones, but up until today, I had thought it was only a girl thing.

"You look like a man on a mission that maybe requires some serious thought," Big Al said to me before I departed. "Have you thought everything through?"

"Yes," I replied.

❖ ❖ ❖

I drove down the road a little farther, several more miles west of the city, traveling past remnants of serenity, fruit and vegetable stands with glimpses of flat open spaces next to pick-up trucks that had wallowed in real dirt. No strip malls or fast food outlets here, the highway was alive with nature and harmony.

I stumbled onto a roadside diner surrounded by oak trees so grand and peaceful they imaged an earlier century. The succulent hamburger was cooked fresh, the outside charred to oblivion and smothered with grilled onions, and for twenty-five cents extra an added glob of authentic Swiss cheese was layered on top. The coffee, thick and tasty and with free refills, was generously offered by the smiling waitress, happy with life, a Spanish-American War widow, loquacious and spry in her support hose-encased legs and geriatric shoes taut with thirty-two inches of laces. The thick rubber soles added to her bounce, but the caffeine rush from her endless supply of coffee spiked my resolve and prompted my pilgrimage to the business at hand.

UB John's Gun Shop and Weapon Emporium resided a mile farther down the road, just as the map predicted, arising quickly like the fog lifting from Brigadoon. It was in a little mall accompanied by an adult book store open twenty-four hours, the fluorescent sign flashing COME OFTEN, and a long-ago shuttered gasoline station displaying a friendly-appearing brontosaurus touting tetraethyl additive and prices that evoked good memories.

It wasn't Gene Kelly or even Van Johnson who greeted me at UB John's—John outweighed them and Big Al by a hundred pounds. No doubt, he was an aficionado of the tasty cheeseburgers up the road at the diner shaded by the grand oaks. There were stocky guys with heads down, adorned with fedoras and dark sunglasses, tenderly fingering the merchandise, interspersed with furtive glances right and left, screening for potential adversaries. They were certainly not the skeet-shooting set, or as we doctors said to one another in the ER about our clients, "they're not the carriage trade."

I didn't need to impress UB John by telling him that Lester M. Gillis and Baby Face Nelson were one and the same, and I didn't inquire as to whether or not he accepted personal checks. When I requested a silencer with the Smith & Wesson .45-caliber semiautomatic pistol, he tendered no lecture about sound-suppression physics or evil consequences. Reaching under the register, he pulled out a shiny metal screw-on device, slapped it on the counter, and waited. UB John could have been the State's purchasing agent approving a road-paving contract. No questions, no eye contact, no bargaining, just a reminder about releasing the safety lever before firing and the added respect when I had requested the silencer.

"Don't forget, if you want to buy in quantity, see me, now that you're a bona-fide UB John customer. Identification is just a routine." Big John winked. It wasn't pretty. He didn't look twice at the Bill Tomczak's driver's license I handed him. There was no special form for the silencer.

Traffic was lighter heading back into the city, going against the early-rush-hour people driving to the blue-collar suburbs. The workers finished at 2 or 3 p.m., the maintenance and cleaning crews, the security people, and the city employees putting in their six-hour day. I hummed out loud. Feeling good and who needed a radio, recalling Erroll Garner fingering the piano keys and grunting while playing "People Will Say We're in Love." Remembering sweet music extracted from recesses deep in your brain is easy when you're happy after a glorious day of acquisitions.

# SIX

I was reading X-rays with the radiologists when Dr. Rhoban paged me. The radiologists held conferences every several hours that were fortified with pleasing refreshments—coffee with coffee aroma and flavor, bakery cakes with layers of frosting and real fruit splayed on top, and a supply of large white paper napkins enclosing authentic plastic forks sealed in cellophane, likely guaranteeing them to be salmonella-free. Twinkies and Hostess Cupcakes were never on the menu.

A VIP professor patient was waiting to see Dr. Rhoban, who was tied up in his laboratory and wouldn't be available for about an hour. If I could start the history and physical examination, Herb would be grateful. Maybe even take it easy on me when I was able to play tennis again.

"Sure," I said, "my pleasure." By now, I was sated with delicacies and barium-enema X-ray pictures.

❖ ❖ ❖

"Hello Professor Bernstein," I said, "I'm Dr. Ted, a medical resident, and Professor, sir, you might remember me." I nervously fingered the stethoscope dangling from around my neck. It was the awkwardness of a student meeting his former professor.

Unless we had been on call the night before, the tradition was to get spiffed up for rotations such as Radiology, with shoelaces of similar color, pristine neckties fastened tight up to the Adam's apple, sleeves that buttoned, and clean shaven faces. I barely recognized myself in my sartorial brilliance; clearly I was stretching my luck hoping for the professor's recollection.

Standing near the writing desk, arms at ease, offering a smile that flashed recognition, he said yes, he remembered me. He appeared the same, although maybe a few pounds lighter. His face was thinner. His suit featured a subtle pattern of quiet blue and gray checks that from a distance merged into a single color, the molded shoulders and chest suggested a facile and expensive tailor. The professor, an eminent dermatologist, was here to see Herb Rhoban in consultation. Usually someone—spouse, child, friend, siblings—accompanied you when you saw Dr. Rhoban. The professor was alone.

"Herb will be here shortly," I informed the professor, "and with your permission, I'll start the examination."

"Explain my fevers and weight loss, will you, and it'll be my pleasure having you as my doctor. Look at me, I've lost ten pounds," he said, while his thumbs pulled the slack between his leather belt and belly.

Where I sit, you hear just about everything, and the professor's symptoms augured nothing good. And everywhere I touched, inspected, pushed, and kneaded—the axilla, the groin, the neck—there were large lymph nodes. The spleen, normally lying quietly beneath the left diaphragm, filled my right hand.

"Professor, thanks for letting me examine you," I said when I completed my assessment, "and thanks for being so cooperative. Be comfortable. Dr. Rhoban and I will be back in a few minutes." Non demonstrative with my words, I could have been reporting summer weather in the Sahara, as I headed to the doctors' station.

With a sweep of my hand, I cleared the writing table of debris, fidgeted down into the swivel chair, rubbed my face a few times, enough to bring pink to my cheeks, closed my eyes, and marshaled my thoughts. Discovering bad things is a doctor's nightmare, and worse was finding it in someone as respected as the professor. The bad tidings recalled memories of my medical school days spent with him.

❖ ❖ ❖

"I'm Dr. Ted, a senior medical student rotating through Dermatology," I'd say to my assigned patient, glossing over the oxymoron, "and I'll examine your rash." The stinginess of the too-short, flimsy paper gown, open in back or front, depending upon the location of the patient's problem, and the room temperature bordering on absolute zero, limited queries regarding my qualifications.

After the briefest of knocks, the professor and his novitiates marched in, the room stuffed like a rush-hour Red Line subway car, but space was always set aside for the professor. "Hello, I'm Dr. Bernstein, and I'm very pleased to make your acquaintance," he announced, snapping his heels ever so slightly, repeating the words to everybody: patient, family, friends, children, all down the line, one by one, like a prince meeting the town folk. And cooing to the babies was not a lost art with the professor.

The professor, closer to sixty than fifty, was a big man, a combination of large bone structure and obesity. A dense, well-groomed crop of black hair towered over protruding eyes and a benign, immobile expression, which remained the same whether he diagnosed syphilis or eczema. His smile was flat, his voice gruff and without variation; he'd diagnose poison ivy, or acne vulgaris, or psoriasis, or herpes zoster after the inspection, his glasses shoved high on his forehead, his face sometimes within an inch or two of the lesion, slowly shaking his head over such aberrations of nature.

And he was open to other opinions.

"Yes, I hear what you're saying," he would say, pointing to the dissenting student or resident. "But believe me when I tell you that this nice person"—hands stroking the patient—"has the most excellent common warts I've come across in years and nothing else. Go ahead and feel the roughness of the lesions and appreciate the normal skin in between."

Dermatology failed a lot of students. I can understand why, but we also performed in desultory fashion in Radiology, Orthopedics, and Ophthalmology, and those departments passed everybody. Our final examination consisted of examining a patient and providing a diagnosis.

My patient was a forty-year-old woman with multiple small, discrete firm nodules, almost on stalks, scattered over most of her body, interspersed with flat brown skin discoloration.

"Doctor," the professor said. An honorific title, as I was not yet a doctor. "What does this nice lady have?" he asked, after he briefly scanned the patient.

"I'm not sure, Professor, I see the pedunculated lesions"—thrilled that I could come up with that term—"and the brown..."

"What does the patient have?" he interrupted, his hands clasped over his abdomen, his eyes fixed on mine. "Please give me the diagnosis, Doctor, or I'll think you've learned nothing in your training with us, and that would greatly disappoint me."

"I'm sorry, Professor, I don't know what the patient has." And I was sorry.

"Tell me, Doctor, do you think the patient has seborrhea?"

I shook my head.

"Could this be atopic eczema?"

"No," I said.

"Is this chicken pox?"

"No," I said again.

"Very good, Doctor. Now tell me what dermatology textbook do you read?"

"*The Modern Textbook of Dermatology*," I offered. How could I go wrong with that fictional choice? None of the students ever read dermatology. The clinic experience with the professor seemed to provide adequate teaching.

"Very good, now reexamine the patient." He directed my gaze down to the bemused lady, who was keenly aware that my predecessors had been more astute. "Read your textbook of dermatology, and you'll learn that this nice lady has classic neurofibromatosis."

❖ ❖ ❖

"You're Polish," the professor told me when we were outside the examining room. There was no admonishment about my diagnostic shortcomings.

"I'm a *yid*," he said" I was Polish once. Our Krakow neighbors helped my family escape the country. I found safety. But not the Poles, they had it tough during and after the War, caught between vengeful armies and then the Russian hegemony. In spite of what they went through, the Poles still struggle for respect. *Yids* and Poles have to prove themselves to the world and to God and be smarter and work harder than others." The professor was speaking to me, eyes smoking in intensity, as if diagnosing a rarity. "Study hard and remember what I just told you—enjoy graduation." And he registered me somewhere in his vast repertoire of memories.

That wasn't the highlight of my medical school career. Did I need the advantage volunteered by the professor? Was it offered to counter the prejudices that other professors had inflicted on minorities, or was it a reflection of the older generation's paranoia? I didn't know the answer, but I was grateful for his gift. And I made amends. I purchased a textbook of dermatology and studied the ins and outs of neurofibromatosis until I could recite the chapter verbatim.

❖ ❖ ❖

The professor was patiently waiting for Dr. Rhoban and me, his glasses settled an inch down on his nose, the paper gown open in back.

Herb doesn't waffle with his medical decisions, and after my presentation and his examination, he offered his opinion. "Lymphoma seems likely," he told the professor without flinching. "Dr. Ted is going to apply several skin tests, one for tuberculosis, and I suggest the lymph node in the right side of the neck be removed for the pathologist."

A quick acquiescence by the professor, and Herb telephoned the surgeon. "Come down to the clinic, introduce yourself to the professor, treat him well, and schedule the biopsy, stat. He'll tell you what lymph node. Good-bye."

It always helps when someone else provides direction for medical problems, especially when it's someone of Herb's stature. The professor had no family around for advice, and he turned to me. "Doctor, did I come in too late? I kept on hoping the symptoms were temporary, like a virus. Some days I'd wake up early, charge out of bed, and feel like my old self again."

"Professor, I'm sure the disease was caught early," I replied. I believed there was no better ministry than the ministry of hope.

"Pray with me," he requested when he had finished, and his fingers reached out for mine.

*Our God and God of all ages,*

*Love us, as much as we will let you.*

*And provide strength and intelligence to me and my Polish friend.*

"Thank you, Doctor," he told me and firmly grasped my hand. "You've come a long way. Congratulations."

I was pleased to receive his commendation and to pray with him. We talked about everyday things until the surgeon arrived.

On my way home, at the S curve facing the lake, snarled in the ebb and flow of the evening rush-hour traffic, my mind became free to wander and I added belatedly, in full voice through the driver's-side window wide open to the heavens: "*Be gracious O Lord, for I have little merit, But please treat the professor generously, and with kindness be his help.*"

# SEVEN

"The coffee's gratis, Sergeant, and same goes for your buddies. Strong men make my heart flutter. I'll toss in two or three strips of bacon at no charge, well, make it two pieces. Have them ask for me, the pretty lady sitting at the register." A coquettish, perpetual-motion Mrs. B was not an appealing sight.

"Good morning, Doctor." She belatedly acknowledged me while glancing at the clock over the entranceway, an angelic smile appearing as if her lottery ticket had just come in. "It's too late to use your on-call coupons," she said.

George rewarded Mrs. B with his earnest smile, mouth stretched wide, teeth flashing, the sergeant always composed, no fidgeting around in the uncomfortable plastic chair. Every locale became his office; we could be debating baseball strategy, or my role as a serial perp, it didn't matter where we were. "I like the attention I get when I come here, the whole hospital actually," he said, hands drumming rhythmically on the tabletop. "Maybe it's not too late for me to apply to medical school. Become a doctor and a smart guy like my good friend Doctor Ted.

"The reason I'm here, Doc," the sergeant continued, maintaining that contented look, no pause for a response from me, "has to do with the beating you took. First, I wanted to see how you're doing, of course. Your good health is my number-one concern, and second, to seek your help in identifying one of Tim Schmidt's enforcers, the guy known on the streets as 'Mr. Baseball.'"

A brief repose, so the sergeant could elevate his coffee cup for Mrs. B's attention for a refill before continuing his discourse, nudging himself closer to me, elbows resting on the table.

"Mr. Baseball spends most of each day at the batting cage, swinging his favorite custom-made lumber at fastballs, curves, out-of-the-strike zone pitches, *bang, bang*, the ball goes a mile. He was a minor league catcher moving up in the system until his manager signaled him to bunt, you know, lay down a sacrifice for the team. But there's no homeruns when you bunt; you're a baseball aficionado, you know that. Right in the dugout, he attacked the unsuspecting manager. Took the whole team, pitchers and all, and you know how effete they are, to get him to stop whacking the manager, for shit's sake. It was his own manager!

"Enforcement is his second career," the sergeant continued. "Generous, he likes to give the unlucky suckers not making the vig a choice in the manner of punishment. And I think he tried honing his stroke on you, Doc."

My sergeant was searching my face and sizing me up for something big, and I began to pay attention.

"Mr. Baseball always asks his victims what joint they want smashed. And depending on his mood, he delivers an on-deck, warmup swing repeated several times, or one homerun cut. He spared you a choice, you probably swore at him or something. Nice guy, huh, and you can't take the Wiffle bat option."

No response from me, the sergeant being on a roll, and his rehash of my encounter with "Mr. Baseball" was riveting in a disaffected way.

"This guy is incorrigible." The sergeant was caught up in his soliloquy and tightening both hands around the handle of the pepper shaker, his own Louisville Slugger, showing me what he considered a major league grip, before continuing his narrative. "I can't get him to offer us information about anything, and get this, Doc, he's here in your hospital, crazy coincidence, huh? Appendicitis at his age, can you believe it?"

Mrs. B stopped by at every lull, refilling the sergeant's coffee, not mine, offering water with ice in a real glass for the policeman, a first for the cafeteria.

"The appendix burst." George loved the attention and didn't miss a beat. "He's receiving antibiotics, getting better too quickly from his surgery, and not seeing the value of confessing his sins. We want you to ID him. It's your chance to get even. Catch him off-guard. We'll give you a wire, just like in the movies. He likes to talk and holds no grudges and you're a Boy Scout to him.

"We don't get too energized when he swings at mob types and the losers failing to meet their weekly payments, but when doctors get beaten up and it's splashed all over the newspapers, we get pressure from the higher-ups to find the perpetrator. After all, as you and I know, we need to make the streets safe for the taxpayers. And as a bonus, if you get any dirt on Tim Schmidt, you'll pass it on."

❖ ❖ ❖

Mr. Baseball was pleased to see me. Infirmity is a lonely journey. His wheelchair placed near the window allowed him glimpses of freedom. The bandages circling his belly were clean. The IV in his arm dripped saline water drop by drop.

"Hey, Doc, I remember you. Nohardfeelingshuh."

No problem deciphering his words now. This was my guy.

"Business is business—right?" Mr. Baseball slowed down his speech for me. "You're the smart one, medicine, good profession, never a recession, always something happening. Look at me, a ruptured appendix at my age. We don't even need the goddamn thing and here I am.

"And look at you, handsome face and no limping. The wiseass fuckers who ask for ankles, they're still limping; they're crips for the rest of their lives. You don't pick up babes when you're a gimp and gimp rhymes with limp. Amazing coincidence, huh? Now all those suckers wish they were smart like you. Always go with the knee."

I didn't tell my new friend that if I could have deciphered his garble back then, I would have chosen the ankle.

This guy was entertaining and motor mouthed like my Clara Barton. I'd have to introduce the two. Stocky, hard, permanent grin, talkative—he'd be considered a catch in some neighborhoods: successful, strong, passably good-looking, except for the hair hiding his knuckles and the encumbrance of the baseball bats.

"Hey, buddy, excuse me for a moment." I turned my back and fussed with the tape recorder slung underneath my white coat, erasing the words already captured and turning off the damn thing. Screw the sergeant. I'm a lot of things, but I'm not a stoolie.

"It's Nikolai V," Mr. Baseball told me, "not to be confused with Nikolai W, and Nikolai Y, my brothers. No Nikolai X, he passed on to a better place."

We shook hands, his other hand holding his belly in, because he couldn't stop laughing. "Same names, everyone Nikolai, crazy family, huh."

With a little luck, I'd never meet them.

"Could you believe my good fortune, when I seen my first baseball game, in a barn of a movie house back in the old country, our Saturday-night entertainment? *The Baby Ruth Story* or some such shit, and I saw this guy, this fat fucker, making wealth, swinging a bat, surrounded by girls, *zaftig* girls. I knew right away America was for me. In my country, swing the beautiful thing and it's off to Siberia."

The hospital gown open in the back, the hem flapping aside with the breeze, the window ajar—windows that opened and closed defined our deluxe suites, fresh air drifting in, or the stale, overheated air out. His fingers worked back and forth, either trying to get a better grip on his imaginary baseball bat or more likely suffering from nicotine deprivation, because he pleaded for a cigarette.

There's no smoking allowed in hospital rooms; everyone knows about the fire hazards associated with the use of 100 percent oxygen. His oxygen tube started from the in-wall tank, extending from its origin above the bed, like a tongue from a fire-breathing dragon, flitting across the floor, looping around his neck, up to his face. The two prongs were loosely inserted into his nostrils and battling for space with exuberant nasal hair, while it *whooshed-whooshed* pure $O_2$.

I lit the cigarette for him. After all, when you come right down to it and scrape away all of the highfalutin pretensions, medicine is a service industry. And half of the doctors smoked. The chief of pulmonary medicine made hospital rounds with a cigarette dangling from his lips, capable of expectorating without removing it. He could have starred on the smoking Olympic team. We knew the stuff was associated with bad tidings, but the information about the terrible impact it had on our health hadn't been officially promulgated by the powers-that-be.

"Hey Nikolai V, who else did you introduce to your bat? Do you clean them after each use? You should, you know, they carry germs. You don't want to be like Typhoid Mary."

He smiled. The only Mary he knew was praised in church on Sundays and holidays.

"Have you tried the new Ted Kluszewski model bat? You'd be happy with its heft." I was talking his talk.

"Doc, Big Klu is one of my favorite guys. He looks great in his White Sox uniform. Polish, he's Polish, you know, like you, great, fucking great, *zajebisty*, and if you want to meet him, let me know. But I order my bats direct from Louisville, my own personal grip, weight, and balance, custom-made for yours truly. You need the perfect balance to feel the *ping* of crushed bones. Grand slams, I call them. Like a wet dream."

Baseball Guy was happier than a dog leaving the vet.

"That's okay, Nikolai V, I just came by to say hello. Big Klu favors aren't needed and I understand the pleasure of swinging the lumber," I said, and pointed out the view from his window, directing his gaze toward the beauty of the downtown skyline lit by the midmorning sun flecked with sparkles bouncing off the skyscraper windows. I pushed the lower pane, the heavy bottom part of the window sash, down on his right hand, like a blunt guillotine made infamous during earlier times in warmhearted France. The hand with the cigarette between his nicotine-stained index and middle finger was now trapped between the window and the sill.

I remembered catching my finger in the car door as a kid. The door completely sealed shut, my father joining me in shedding tears, while struggling to pry it open—the pain indelibly fixed in my long-lived memory neurons.

I had to give Nikolai V credit. I wondered whether his brothers would be as stoic. No whining, just: "*Enough, enough, Doc, enough, openthedamnwindow*."

His fingers were crushed and angry-looking, as I pried the window open, freeing his hand, then unlocking his wheelchair and pushing him toward the sink. The oxygen cord popping free from the wall, trailed us like a thin green garden snake wriggling toward home. Nikolai V held his damaged hand high, a good first aid maneuver, because elevating injured body parts limited the swelling by reducing the blood supply.

"Goodness, Nicky, such an unfortunate happening, the window coming down on your fingers like that. One would think that couldn't happen in a hospital of all places. I'll be sure to notify the hospital safety officer."

"Quick, Doc, get the cold water running. This is big-time pain." Once again, Nikolai V impressed me with the breadth of his medical knowledge, as I turned on the hot water faucet. That was another issue I'd take up with the safety officer; our hot water was almost boiling temperature. It's okay if you want instant tea or coffee, but it was not exactly therapeutic for crushed fingers.

I held my friend's hand in the near-boiling water for just five seconds. It probably seemed longer.

"Nikolai V, not Nick, thanks for not screaming or pushing the call button for help. You've restored my faith in machismo. No hard feelings, either. Business is business."

I told the charge nurse about the unfortunate accidents that had taken place in room 427 as I left the floor.

I informed the sergeant that I wasn't sure about the identity of the patient. "I didn't obtain any helpful information except for his brothers' first names, Nikolai and Nikolai," I mumbled, as I returned the tape recorder.

"You see," I told the sergeant, "I have trouble identifying even the major leaguers. Minor leaguers are beyond me, especially when they're hitting me."

Nikolai V and I were even. Street justice had rules, and I had adopted them.

# EIGHT

The IntMed 3s taught Physical Diagnosis, called "p-dog" in the vernacular, to the second-year medical students. This was the students' first hands-on patient experience. We obtained histories and performed physical examinations on hospitalized patients willing to submit to our questions and probing fingers. I had a reputation for being a good teacher, and I felt I was accomplishing something good. I routinely used humor to cover my inadequacies; it was ingrained in me. My father used to test me by mixing facts with absurdities: "Is it colder in the winter or in Chicago?" he'd ask.

A single heart murmur, or one swollen lymph node, or an enlarged spleen or liver in an articulate patient, facilitated our learning. Finding these teaching gems required snooping around the hospital floors and cajoling the patients into allowing the five of us, the four students and me, to take up their afternoon and amateurishly poke around their psyche and body. The funny thing was, though, most patients enjoyed participating in the teaching exercise and graciously shared their time and energy with us. I think for the infirm, the youth and freshness of the students ignited an affirmation of life.

Sharon, the brightest of the four students, two women and two men, obtained the histories, while we sat around observing her technique. This was our second go-around of medical history procurement and I wanted the exercise to be challenging.

Mrs. Kessler had difficulty focusing her thoughts. Elderly and frail, but bright-eyed, eager, and pleased for our company, she shook Sharon's hand and invited her to sit next to her, while we found chairs and surrounded her hospital bed.

"I'm Sharon, Mrs. Kessler, a second-year medical student, and I would like to ask you some questions about the reason for your hospitalization."

"Well, I'm here because they brought me to this place, dear," Mrs. Kessler responded. Women in medicine didn't receive much respect and were seldom called doctors. "And I'd like to go home. My stay here has been a pleasant one, thank you. Would you please call me a taxi?"

Sharon looked at me, I smiled back and encouraged her to continue, my hands placed out flat in front of me like the umpire's safe call. No one had promised that medicine was easy.

"Mrs. Kessler,"—Sharon turned back to her—"I don't mean to be rude in asking these questions, but do you know where you are and what day it is?"

*Good going, Sharon, asking the right questions, assessing the patient's mental status.*

"Isn't this my home? John, my husband, let you in, didn't he? What a rascal he is for not telling me."

John was long dead.

"And what was your other question, dear? Oh, I remember now, it's Thursday or whatever day of the week and you're going to ask me to subtract 7 from 100, and ask me who's the mayor, aren't you? Well it's Mayor Daley."

Mrs. Kessler had it down pat.

I thanked Mrs. Kessler for her time and we gathered in the conference room down the hall. Bert was pissed that we'd spent time with this frail lady, instead of hearing about acute gallbladder or pneumonia symptoms. A surgeon-in-waiting, he reveled in the histories of painful or blocked organs. Ron, as usual, was silent. I had difficulty fathoming his perceptions. The prototypic IntMed candidate, skinny, nearsighted, he dissected the important medical information I provided, and pointed out the discrepancies. Quiet at the bedside, I couldn't intimidate him with my stares. Phyllis, our fourth student, smiled somewhat aimlessly, participated wordlessly, dressed too formally for our work—nail polish, tight skirts, and frilly blouses looked good under a newly acquired white coat, but her outfits were too formal for the knock-down dirty life of a medical student. She would change.

Sharon smiled at me. "I know how much time you spend selecting patients for us. You asked us to see Mrs. Kessler for a reason, didn't you?"

"Of course I did. This exercise has a purpose," I answered. "When Mrs. Kessler frustrates us because we can't understand what her medical problems are after asking our standard questions, we must think about illnesses just as important as heart or kidney disease. Think memory loss, delirium, or confusion. Poor Mrs. Kessler has dementia and possibly schizophrenia and she needs our understanding."

I didn't convince everybody, but Mrs. Kessler reinforced the complexities of medicine.

Other lessons were less dramatic, listening to heart murmurs, and percussing the chest and the heart border might have been more fun, but Mrs. Kessler played on our minds and Sharon paid her a daily visit.

Pelvic and rectal examinations were taught by the gynecology department. We were responsible for everything else. Ear canals and lymph nodes were easy. It was the scrotal examinations that were challenging. How do you tactfully ask a patient to agree to allow four young students to palpate his testes and prostate?

"Hello sir, I'm Dr. Ted. How are you today? Oh, I'm sorry to hear that—we hope you'll feel better real soon. I wonder if it would be okay if we examine your privates. I'm sure you won't mind."

And most of the time they didn't.

Strange isn't it?

My group handled the course exceptionally well. They described heart murmurs they heard rather than what I told them.

"Hear the soft, holosystolic murmur with the snapping second sound," I said, while I handed them my stethoscope turned to mute.

"Dr. Ted, I'm not hearing anything," they told me.

We paid a visit to Mrs. Stone. She and I hugged. She was recovering from stomach surgery. There was a malignant growth there. The Virchow's node finding was accurate. Some dicta in medicine are almost always correct, and that was one of them. Rudolf Virchow, himself, called the node named after him "the seat of the devil."

Mrs. Stone was receptive to the students' questions and she recounted her medical history for them. It was their first encounter with a patient with a malignancy, and the poignancy of the inevitable would unfortunately be diluted with repetition.

The students often showed up on nights when I was on call. Medicine was the most challenging then. Decisions required amalgamation of the history, the physical examination, and bedside intuition—plus the technology of the laboratory and the X-ray clues. At that moment in time, the scope of our profession seemed boundless—and the students' questions and enthusiasm boded well for the future of medicine.

# PART FOUR

# ONE

## *Early Spring 1962*

Tim Schmidt's office was close to the hospital and easy to find. The narrow commercial streets were well-marked and straight. Diagonal avenues bisecting our city at odd angles and screwing up one's mental compass spared this area. I found a parking space tagged with a parking meter accepting dimes that sometimes provided sixty minutes of respite and sometimes nothing. The arbitrariness was supported by its malicious grin pantomiming: "*feed me, feed me*." This old, inbred enclave had parking enforcers who would only ticket outsiders, although my decrepit car fit in well.

The city's vaunted, but slow "rapid" transit line was a city block away. Climb about one-hundred steps, no help for the infirm, and you could travel north or south, the former direction setting me down near my apartment. Indiana, $35^{th}$, Chinatown, Roosevelt, Harrison, Jackson and Adams and I was downtown. The screech of the metal wheels stopping and accelerating on the shiny metal tracks embedded in the dark wood, elevated structure provided background syncopation for the neighborhood symphony.

Rather nondescript, it was a one person office, heralded only by a stenciled sign in the window with Tim Schmidt's name and the eponymous INSURANCE. No neon daggers or hacksaws flickering on and off in alternating rhythm. The office, nestled in a block of small retail stores: a budget women's shoe store, nothing fancy, mostly black, low-heeled, and with laces, a beauty salon, a Lithuanian bakery, the window stacked with freshly baked pumpernickel; the family businesses topped with residential apartments populated by the white ethnic, Eastern European population. Hardworking citizens all, loyal, stoic, with strong ties to their homelands, they distrusted outsiders and remained content with the status quo. The Moody Bible Institute kids and the Lubavitchers didn't proselytize here.

My working-class clothes and scruffy looks were an asset as I strolled around the neighborhood, no eye contact, surveying the community and getting my bearings straight for the business at hand. No stopping for a shot and beer chaser and sports playing on the bulky television set fastened high above the bar at the taverns gracing every corner; no arguing balls and strikes with the owner and the retirees and the out-of-work residents.

Occasionally the stars and planets align favorably. Tim left his office without locking the door behind him, looking neither left nor right, and why not? This was his turf. Who would dare break into his office, while he walked east toward a restaurant featuring *HOME COOKING by Mrs. Rose* printed on both large windows that were dark and streaky with condensation and bare except for the signs. A popular spot, in spite of its humble appearance, customers flowed in and out crowding the small vestibule made narrower with the city and neighborhood newspaper dispensers. Tim, as big and surly-appearing as I remembered, strode forcefully into the diner and through the doors, no one obstructing his way.

I hustled back to my car and retrieved my .45-caliber, semiautomatic pistol topped with the silencer enclosed in a brown paper bag. The package resembled the sacks that alcoholics caress when surreptitiously sipping their liquid lifeline while sitting on a street curb or a deserted park bench.

I boldly walked into Tim's office, right into his space, past a waiting room with two clean and newer tan-colored, cushiony sofas with reading material stacked in between. *Road and Driver*, *Hunting and Fishing*, that ilk; there were no *New Yorkers* or *Consumer Reports*. I now knew what to send Tim for Christmas if my plan failed. I placed my brown paper bag offering under his desk, snug between the bottom unstained wood-fiber paneling and the plush high-pile gray carpet the color of factory smoke, covering the entire floor. My package, hidden from view from the casual visitor, would hopefully remain undisturbed, away from the cleaning lady, or Tim's prying eyes searching the floor for dropped greenbacks or a severed ear.

I left for home, not wanting to stay around the neighborhood or even be near Tim's office until later, when the sky would darken. I fantasized that my package contained an explosive I could trigger while kneeling at St. Stanislaus praying for Betty's soul—my recitations triggering the thing. But no, I really didn't wish that, not at all. I was greedy; I wanted personal touches with my vendetta.

Thoughts of revenge created a hunger, and I prepared my special peanut butter and jelly sandwich to be washed down with a Coke. Crunchy peanut butter, extra-thick, applied generously on weeks-old Wonder Bread, the speckled, white mold discoloration hidden by an application of a thin layer of cream cheese, the same color as the fungus. The cream cheese supplement, my own creation, supplied additional cholesterol and fat calories to the delicacy while also adding extra smoothness.

Tim answered after the first telephone ring.

"Doctor, what a surprise!" seemingly not surprised at all. "I can't say it's a pleasant one, but heck, if you need health or life insurance, maybe I can help you out. Although, Doctor, after seeing your face in the newspapers after the beating—such a tragic occurrence by the way but I'm sure an instructive one—I'd have to increase the premiums. You seem to be accident-prone. Buy term insurance. It's cheaper than whole life, and by the way, I have a friend recovering from appendicitis and a sore hand who sends you his greetings.

"What can I do for you?" Tim's voice was fading, his enthusiasm dissipated after the insurance man's spiel and gossip.

"Give your friend my best, and of course my best to you," I said. "Tim, I have some information about Betty's death I want to share with you. No insurance purchase right now, but many thanks for the info. Something new has come up about Betty, and I need to talk to you about it, before talking to the police. How about meeting me this afternoon or early evening?"

We agreed. Just the two of us. I volunteered that I was taking the train and would be off work at 5 p.m., and I would leave then.

I drove and circled the area a few times, then parked between the station and Tim's office. No one carrying a bat stood sentry near the entrance. A Cubs hat sat snug on my head. Not cool. This was a White Sox stronghold; the Cubs were the enemy. I would discard the thing as soon as possible. People would notice it, and I had never owned or worn one in my life—my grand attempt at disguise.

I carried a small cloth gym bag with wide brown and black stripes, a faded *St. Michael's* SAC printed on both sides, and a worn leather handle. Trim dark sunglasses were plastered to my face, and tired jeans and a sweater, the latter either dark blue or black, it was difficult to tell the difference in the late afternoon.

Tim was in charge as we patted one another down. Routine for him, we were first-time lovers groping one another, hands on chests, back pockets, and upper thighs. He carefully inspected my gym bag, finding a few paperback mystery books, a notepad and writing paper.

"Doc," he told me after our fondling, "such wonderful publicity you received after that baseball bat encounter. You could open an office and advertise as the famous doctor, the beaten-up, but-not-too-badly, famous doctor. The stories and photos plastered in your waiting room would provide better credentials than a Purple Heart."

Punctured lung and fractured patella weren't considered too harsh—I suppose, in Tim's world, surviving that beating built character and provided entré into his club.

"Doc," he enthused, "let's go to some ballgames together, play racquetball at the club, and down a six-pack of cold Schlitz to cool off. Sometimes I buy, sometimes you do, but just one piece of advice— you'll have to change hats. Not too many Cubs fans around here."

I nodded. I was simply a passenger.

"We'll take in a Blackhawk game, beat up some skinny guys in suits, take their girls, and really bond. My guess is, we'd have a lot of laughs. What do you think?"

Smiling, blue-collar, sociable Tim, successful insurance agent, verbose, this was his other side, perhaps only alcohol released his furies. We stared at one another, neither wanting to blink first. Him at his desk, the doc sitting across in a comfortable faux-leather chair with molded arms covered with the same plastic material, smiling, good old guys talking about fun times, but deep down, we remained bitter enemies. His anger and our competitiveness were on the verge of erupting, as if anticipating another fifteen minutes of hard-fought basketball or football. North Side versus South Side, blue-collar versus middle-class aspirations, different schools and neighborhoods, the Catholic League Youth Championship on the line, neither of us daring to lose. Nothing held back. Handshakes offered only because they were required.

"Tim, one of the nurses returned to work and she wanted my advice about the events surrounding Betty's death. She noticed something unusual on that night." My fabricated story was well-rehearsed. "For the moment I told her not to go to the police."

"What the shit are you talking about? Betty's dead," Tim shouted, now out of control, happening quickly as he levitated from his chair, his words showering spit. "Betty's *dead*. A loser, sick, sick all the time, she's in a better place, only it would've been *mucho* better if some wiseass doctor didn't have her all carved up for nothing and then foist the police on me." After a pause, the fidgeting stopped, his cool returning as quickly as his tirade began, he leaned forward on his desk, resting on his elbows, making certain I was paying attention. "Don't try to pin her death on me, you can't," he said, a thick index finger pointed my way. "I read the autopsy report. My lawyer got me a copy. And just like what I told you, she died of lupus."

"Tim?" I asked, now more confident after watching him explode, his eyes rolling around, never in the same place, just like they did the night at the hospital. "Confess to me that you killed Betty. I need the closure. I can't sleep at night, thinking it was me who failed to treat her. It won't go anywhere. I promise. Cross my heart." And just like back in schooldays when the fifth-graders made promises, I crossed my heart, my right hand making two diagonals over my chest. "Just as you said, Tim, nothing can implicate you. Do that and I'll forget what the nurse told me. What do those busybody, constantly chattering, foreign nurses know anyway?" I drew nearer, head leaning forward like we were conspirators. “Maybe you’d even be willing to share some of Betty’s life insurance with me.”

“Doctor, all of a sudden we’re talking the same language. I like your attitude.” No change in Tim’s expression, but there was just a hint of a laugh. “I won’t admit to nothing, there’s nothing in it for me until you tell me what you have.” Tim was back to business. Smart.

Photographs of him smiling hung behind his head on the back wall, black-and-whites, neatly fixed on a poster board with merrily colored plastic-capped pins securing the golf outings, insurance conventions, and deep-sea fishing on the stern of a generous sized yacht, miles of calm blue sea surrounding him. Tim hoisting a beer in the backyard with scary looking buddies the size of NFL offensive linemen celebrating some nefarious deed. Where were the photos of Tim beating his wife or tweaking the noses of people short of cash on the due date?

“Tim, I’m going to reach into my gym bag and retrieve my pad of paper with the information I want to give you.”

Tim killed Betty. All the time I had spent in his office and I didn’t hear one denial.

I rustled down around my feet, making no sudden moves, providing Tim with a narrative of my actions, while I pushed the gym bag aside and reached under the desk for my brown paper bag, fussing around on the floor, as if I’d dropped something.

And finding nothing!

“Oops,” I cleverly whispered, as I knelt down on my hands and knees, searching for my precious package. Maybe Tim had discovered it because I had placed it too close to his big feet and soon I’d be a dead duck.

“What the fuck are you doing down there?” Tim demanded, back in charge of the world but speaking without anger. His gigantic black shoes were still planted on the carpet underneath the desk, the carpet less worn there, a thicker and deeper shade of gray and the color unsullied by body fluid.

“You don’t have to clean there, Doc, I pay an overpriced service to do that and if I’d wanted my shoes polished, I’d have told you.” A verbose and relaxed Tim talking.

Miss Sheehy, my fourth grade teacher, would place the bad boys under her desk as punishment for misbehavior. I became familiar with the smell of feet and shoes and the body odor of middle-aged teachers blessed with perverted ideas of discipline. But there was light at the end of this tunnel, because my brown paper bag sat a little farther back and just inches in front of Tim's cordovans. The gun with the silencer in place was as long and hefty as the mail-order Red Ryder BB rifle that accompanied my preadolescence. The latter's purchase gobbled up a year of allowance savings and Oh Henry! and Butterfinger candy-bar sacrifices, and then I was never allowed to use it.

My pistol was completely wrapped with a new invention, Saran plastic wrap, polymerized plastic that clung to everything. Discovered by error—think penicillin, LSD and other miracles—it nicely enveloped my deadly cannon-like contraption. I didn't need gloves. There'd be no Dr. Ted fingerprints on this pistol, and the silencer purchased from UB John's would minimize the commotion.

I stood up, gun in my right hand, clumsily extracting the thing from the brown paper bag, my left hand propping up the barrel. The bag stuck between my fingers. The weapon felt cool in my hand, the term "carrying "heat" was imprecise. I held the thing firm like a baby robin being hoisted back into the nest. Calm and collected, even though this was all new to me, since the last gun I'd fired propelled darts tipped with rubber suction cups that always failed to stick.

Shit! There was a family picture of Tim on the desk. I hadn't noticed it. The two cute kids Betty had shown me, the older girl with her arm around her brother, both with the artificial smiles children generate when thinking mayhem, squinting at the camera, standing next to the stern patriarch and a smiling Betty. The latter's eyes on her spouse. He was a family man frolicking in his backyard on a peaceful weekend day. Just to their side was a large silver-colored, rectangular metal, charcoal grill, smoke enveloping the bratwursts precisely lined up, one by one over the coals, a family scene that reminded me so much of the photograph hanging in my bedroom.

My father once came home with a borrowed German camera, small, shiny, metallic gray, precise-appearing with a lens that slowly moved forward and back with a twist of your fingers, and a long metal cable hanging down, all sitting on a bulky tripod. "Picture-taking time," he announced, while fussing over its placement as we stood on our back porch, next to the grill, the same brand as Tim's, but Polish sausages cooking, not bratwursts. "Ten beeps accompanied by tiny red flashes," Father said, pressing the starter button, then running around to join Mother and me as we counted, laughing at each sound, "*eight, nine, ten*"—and the camera clicked and the lens opened wide on cue. The three of us recorded for posterity, very handsome, the camera liked us, a five-by-seven black-and-white, framed, and the date plainly written on the bottom in soft pencil.

I looked Tim in the eyes and for a smart, tough dude in a mean business for many years he didn't seem to have a clue as to what was happening. No fear pulling his face. I think his unwariness reflected his confidence. After all, what could happen to him in his own private office, on this ordinary day, with this mild-mannered young doctor who just a moment ago was groveling at his feet and was now carrying a mélange of brown paper bag, plastic wrap, and a metal tube that was held in two palsied hands?

Tim was blown backward. He hit hard against the wall containing the photographs, knocking down the eighteenth-golf-hole print, the one with Tim's smile directed at the camera, just after putting out a winning round, as evidenced by his happy look, ready to cash in on his wagers, the frame and picture still upright and facing frontward, lying below the new hole in his upper chest.

I had aimed at his belly, remembering the writhing of victims after receiving "gut shots" in the action movies I'd absorbed as a kid, and not at his face, trying to show a little civility. But the recoil of the pistol had jerked the weapon upward toward the chest. The noise was moderate like several ceramic plates breaking, or a stack of newspapers falling to the ground, but the power and the simplicity of the destruction was overwhelming.

Blood seeped onto Tim's carpet. He should have had a mat or throw rug there. "*Clean up the blood with cold water, it works better than solvents, and warm water won't touch it*," I wanted to tell him. Gangsters wouldn't know that.

I would need to get rid of my clothes with the stink of the nitrites, but the Saran Wrap, wonder of wonders, remained intact. Kudos to the inventors. I wanted to hear a confession, but heard nothing other than a buzz bouncing inside my ears. Tim's eyes glazed over too quickly for me to ask what Mozart or Puccini aria the angels were humming to accompany his Act of Contrition. I had seen enough dying in my young career, only a few my doing, none so dramatic, and I wasn't going to call a Code-One. It wouldn't have helped.

I declined Tim's offer for term insurance, replaced the gun into the versatile brown paper sack and lowered it into my gym bag. Brushing off the top of the desk with my handkerchief, I tidied up, turned the family picture facedown, switched off the lights, and prepared to leave. I didn't need souvenirs, my memories would suffice. Careful to not touch anything else in the office, I checked Tim's schedule book on his desk and ripped a page off. There was no mention of meeting the doc.

Nobody was knocking on the door. No passersby coming to call, no clients paying their weekly premium. No hit men strolling in to report their successes, while the sky darkened and the neighborhood stores began to slow their pace before closing.

I felt better. Even at peace. I pulled my Cubs cap down over my head, sunglasses, snug in place, while I carefully let myself out of the office, wiping the door knob with my handkerchief. No one was around, the street nearly deserted. I hoped Tim had enough life insurance himself and wondered whether it was whole life or his favorite, a term policy. Tim had been a father, a husband, a son, and there would be sadness—his catafalque, the bloodied office chair. It could have been different.

Heading toward the train station, making no eye contact with the commuters, I entered the enclosed train lobby, doors swinging in rhythm with the departing passengers, and dumped Tim's appointment sheet with today's schedule on top of the trashcan near the door. The gun stayed with me, resting gently in my gym bag.

Turning around, I joined the flow of tired workers heading home and walked toward my car. No parking ticket on the window, the tires still inflated, the engine turned over, General Motors was the best, their cars started reliably. It was the rust, like gangrene, that would eventually spoil my automobile.

No middle finger flashed to the drivers of the expensive cars not equipped with turn signals. I was mellow and drove carefully, not needing an altercation or accident or traffic ticket. My anger receptors were sated from the afternoon's activity. I understood why gangsters and hit men spent so much of their time relaxing at spas and health clubs on their off days.

I arrived at River Park, an underused city forest on the northwest side adjacent to the Chicago River's North Branch, and slipped on my sleek White Sox black satin jacket and running shoes stored in the trunk. I removed the Saran Wrap from my .45-caliber avenger and discarded it, only to cover the pistol with more of the stuff—the fingerprints present on the handle needed to be preserved. They were my safety net.

Carrying the splendid pistol on its last journey, snug in the familiar brown bag, I became a late-afternoon jogger running toward the river, stopping only once at a bench lining the path to tie my shoelaces tight. In my nervousness, I hadn't pulled the shoestrings taut like good runners always do. Clumsiness now, tripping and falling over dangling laces and triggering my pistol to action, would be dumb.

I threw my special package into the brine, watching it sink quickly and unlike *My Darling Clementine,* it was gone, but maybe not forever. Carefully triangulating its watery grave, I would record the landmarks when I arrived home. "Good-bye, my friend, and thanks," I said. Talking aloud to inanimate objects was important in lessening tension.

The run back to the car was pleasantly uncomplicated. I drove toward home and stopped at the park closer to my neighborhood, no river there, the evening light just about drained from the heavens. I ran several times around the composition track in an eccentric route of my own making, smiling, nodding, and talking to the joggers enjoying their own after-work and before-dinner release of frustrations. I leaped high in the air to retrieve the rapidly ascending helium balloons lost by crying children fresh from a birthday party, none of them listening to their parents about securely holding onto them. Personable me, someone would remember my happy face if I needed a timetable of my whereabouts.

And then home to dispose of my clothes and the dreaded baseball hat in a neighbor's trashcan. They would be collected tomorrow. The running gear tossed in its usual spot in the closet, a long shower, the hot water beating down hard and relaxing my muscles, tense from the afternoon's activities. The gunpowder residual slid down the drain along with any lingering doubts surrounding my undertaking.

The nourishment provided from a can of cold SpaghettiOs, with the remaining stale Wonder Bread coated with butter, employed to sop up the liquid red stuff remaining on the sides and bottom of the can, restored my blood sugar and spirits. Violence creates a large appetite. I'll recommend it to my anorexics. After devouring the tasty little Os and washing down the dinner treat with a glass of cold milk, I was off to bed.

I should have slept the slumber of the innocent, because it was about Betty and my knee and my lung, and it was about what was right and fair and correct in our civilized world. Winston Churchill once said, "Nothing is more costly, nothing is more sterile than vengeance." He was wrong.

But why did the wind that rushed down from our lake and spin through the hollows of the city and seep underneath the narrow space below my bedroom window, chill my soul to the core, as if the devil lusted for my warmth? Was it at all possible, I said to myself, for the Lord in his generous love to lift a veil and understand my actions?

❖ ❖ ❖

Howard called with the news. It was 6:30 a.m. Tim Schmidt had been found murdered, gangland-style, sitting at his desk. Justice had been served.

The first-page column in the morning newspaper reported that a prominent insurance salesman with gang ties had been found shot dead, along with information about his connections, and speculation that he had angered some of them. The newspapers sadly noted the two young orphaned children he left behind, accompanied by a photograph of them stoically fighting off tears while standing with an aunt and uncle who talked about a good man dying young.

People die all the time. Leaders, innovators, scientists, philosophers, soldiers, and yet the headlines this day were about Tim, the wife-beater and gangster.

"MURDERER ON CITY EL TRAIN" was plastered on the front page of the afternoon edition. Hopefully the rest of the news was more accurate. How wonderful the headlines would read if I had taken the train home and had been harassed by some goofballs until I pulled out the .45-caliber with ammunition to spare, my enforcer still warm to the touch, and wasted them for society's benefit.

George Esposito paged me, and before I could wonder what the hospital operators thought about my recurring police connections, George asked whether I had heard the news about Tim. No "Doc" or "Ted," he was Sergeant George Esposito calling and I was Dr. Shluzkinski.

"Where were you late yesterday afternoon, when Tim Schmidt was killed?" he asked in a neutral, no-nonsense voice.

"George, on my early day"—he was still George to me—"I slept, exercised, read the funnies, kept-up-to date with *Li'l Abner* and the wonderful Schmoos. I bet if you politely, but firmly, ask those cute dumplings for help, they'd solve some of the more difficult cases for you." No laughter from the sergeant.

I mentioned the late-afternoon jog where I'd gone, and the people I'd spread good tidings to, and added, "And just like you, Sergeant, on a free afternoon, I open a can or two of brewski, work on my oatmeal cookie recipe for the Pillsbury Bake-Off, and play Old Maid until my fingernails dry, and, yes, I was alone."

It became sticky when he asked me whether I owned a handgun, but I had rehearsed that answer, too, and was somewhat truthful.

"George, after my beating, I purchased a pistol. You know you can't be too careful these days. Being a doctor, the dealers and addicts always think you're carrying drugs or loads of cash and they'll try anything to relieve you of them. A person has to protect himself."

"What kind of gun did you purchase, Doctor?" There was no joy resonating in George's voice.

"I don't know what kind. I bought what they sold me—they're all about the same, aren't they?" I answered.

There was silence. I think that the detective didn't want to know more. The questioning had started out as part of the routine murder investigation of Tim Schmidt, and the sergeant had been hoping I had been hard at work on the day of the murder and that doctors never purchase handguns.

# TWO

Months merge into one another when you're a medical resident. You never see the outside. The sudden downpours and the ice storms only become topics of conversation. No snow angels are splayed on top of pristine powder, no snowballs shaped with pebbles inside are tossed at your many enemies. The balmy season offers nothing but leftovers. I stepped outside and it was dark, the parking lot empty, freezing rain and the falling barometer hitting me like a sledgehammer, and I was wearing a summer windbreaker.

❖ ❖ ❖

The Medicine Consultation Service clears patients in the morning, so they can undergo surgery. Fees from the operating rooms are the cash-cow that drives the hospital. We read the electrocardiograms and declare no ischemia, lower the blood sugar with quick-acting insulin, treat the hypokalemia with 20 milli-equivalents of potassium chloride added to the intravenous infusions, and send the patients off on their way.

There was time in the afternoon to linger over coffee. The back tables of the cafeteria at the blind spot belonged to us, our voices the only intrusion as we grumbled about life, the institution, our schedules, and similar irritants that continued *ad infinitum*, until one Wednesday midday, the neurology service asked us to see Mrs. Collins. Surgery was not in her forecast but her doctors needed help with the diagnosis.

A handsome and successful mother and wife, Mrs. Collins was slipping into dementia while her family wrung their hands, bemoaning her fate and medicine's ineptitude. Memory loss, muscle weakness, confusion, and spastic gait were never good developments.

And all the laboratory tests were normal, the family was told.

I sat close, the side rail lowered, our heads inches apart; my chair snug up to her bed so I could hear her soft-spoken responses. Beribboned clay flower pots trumpeting broad green leaves vied for breathing space with a holiday of freshly cut annuals. Their rainbow hues struck a false gaiety and their scent masked the waft of decay.

"Doctor, do you smoke?" Mrs. Collins asked, lying at attention, molded by crisp hospital sheets. She grabbed my hand, her fingers long and graceful, and her thick gray head of hair exuberant in spite of her travails.

"No, I don't smoke and I make it a rule to not provide cigarettes to patients, no matter how regal their presence," I answered.

"Good," she replied, "because terrible things happen to me when I smoke or when someone smokes around me, and when I tell my family and doctors about it they laugh, shake their heads, and snort in disbelief."

I was listening, but not very carefully. I had heard just about everything there was in medicine.

"I go blind!" And she repeated it more emphatically: "*I go blind*! Is there anything crazier than that?" Tears navigated down her cheeks. "Even when smoke is blown at me or when entering a smoky room, the same thing happens. I can't see!"

In all my working years I had heard every complaint from the bizarre to the sad. At times, I became a Bozo the Clown punching bag, my head nodding back and forth saying "uh-huh, uh-huh, uh-huh" but I had never heard about smoke causing blindness before, and I pulled myself straighter in the plastic chair, my interest piqued.

"That does sound strange, Mrs. Collins, but not crazy. Cigarette smoke makes you blind!" I repeated her words. "Thanks for telling me. I'll try to find an explanation for that, and if one exists, I'll find it. That's what I do."

"You're not like the other people here, are you, Doctor?" she asked, pointing around the empty room with a shaky index finger. "They're imposters. Why my family brought me here, I don't know. My eldest son, it's not really him.

"Did you see the movie *The Invasion of the Body Snatchers*? That's what's happening here—people aren't who they seem to be."

Every scene of that black-and-white classic was imprinted in my memory. The good doctor, Miles J. Bennell, played by Kevin McCarthy, elevated himself to stardom as he investigated the strange happenings in Santa Mira. The final kiss, colder even than deep space, with the brand-new alien Becky Driscoll, still resonated in my dreams.

Gentle prodding kept Mrs. Collins awake while I completed the examination. The abnormalities in the unlucky lady could fill a neurology textbook: hyperactive reflexes, loss of vibration sense, up-going toes, spastic pointing—her index finger wandering away to her ear when I asked her to touch her nose.

❖ ❖ ❖

"Give me a few minutes," Ursula, the chief medical librarian, sighed as she left the library, fiddling with her door keys, about to lock up her office. She resided at the opposite end of the pole of her snappish coworkers who harangued me about leaving the stacks in a mess, or about a journal's index pages fused together with Wrigley's Doublemint gum. Resigned to my brashness, Ursula knew complaining was pointless. Her children awaiting her homecoming were old enough to heat their own supper. She returned to her office, spread her coat precisely across the back of her swivel chair, wriggled in next to the index card files, and started searching for answers.

Truth was, I've always been a wiseguy, and the worst kind, one frequently with correct answers. I chose to believe I made this institution a better place. I made eye contact and spoke knowingly, emphasizing points with my fist striking my open palm, so that most of the time I got away with my attitude.

❖ ❖ ❖

"Dr. Stiller, it's Dr. Ted, a medical resident." Dr. Stiller was the chief of ophthalmology and I was telephoning him at home. "I'm attending a patient who becomes blind when exposed to cigarette smoke," I told him, "and I know you're an expert about that." Who knew, maybe he was.

Dr. Stiller must have read the same articles that Ursula had placed in front of me. I nodded thanks to her and flashed an unseen thumbs-up to Dr. Stiller.

❖ ❖ ❖

"Dr. Frank Zitfield speaking, how may I help you?" The same question, whether it was the White House on the line, or me, the flunky assigned to the consultation service. Frank was the chief of the service and the most thorough and friendliest of the successful downtown doctors. I would have loved to work with him in his private office after graduation if he would ask me. He hadn't.

Frank agreed to host a combined meeting between the neurologists and our team for the following morning. Always a competitive get-together, these inter service conferences mimicked the roller derby and the AWA wrestling that blared on the cafeteria's television set.

The morning of our event began with great promise; the city was cold, clear, and sunny. Lake Michigan lies vertical, like a lavaliere touched by gravity, with the hospital and the entire city for that matter clinging to its bottom left. The mountain of clouds building high over the lake would swoop in later and bring rain.

The chief of neurology, short in stature, natty, and self-assured, told us about the abnormalities detected on Mrs. Collins's examination. "It mimics the combined disease of the spinal cord so characteristic of pernicious anemia." But then he added with a sardonic smile, "Challenge number one: the patient," He said "patient," referring to Mrs. Collins in the third person, making her inanimate, distancing himself from her, a maneuver we all used when we were uncertain about the diagnosis and the patient's health was deteriorating.

"The patient," he repeated, "doesn't have anemia, and her red blood cells are normal in shape, and these abnormalities are always found in pernicious anemia," he said with just the right amount of professional concern, standing in front of the blackboard, lecturing to the uninformed.

The room, one of the snug conference rooms attached to every nursing floor, was crowded with house staff, students, and attending doctors. Ledges became bleacher seats, skin stuck to white plastic office chairs, the light was thickly filtered by accumulated dirt, the windows having last been washed in a previous even-numbered year. Stale doughnuts, tepid coffee, and spilled cream littered the long, centrally placed, and deeply scarred wooden table piled with outdated laboratory results, and sullied with both strawberry and KY jelly.

The consult team was prepared.

"It's called tobacco amblyopia, or blindness caused by cigarette smoke," Dr. Zitfield murmured, almost a whisper, catching everyone's attention, and coupled with a practiced pause. In his crisp, charcoal-gray suit, fresh from the dry cleaners, snug in the waist and three-buttoned, he could have been the poster boy for the American Medical Association. Doctors like him were at the vortex of attention, their opinions solicited and respected, their jokes repeated and their stories uninterrupted.

"I'm sure you all picked up on that," he continued. Of course, only we knew about it, and thanks to Ursula and the chief of ophthalmology we were experts. I added credence to our surprise diagnosis, distributing articles about this strange happening when nicotine exposure causes ocular vasoconstriction and temporary blindness.

"Even high school graduates"—it was my turn to expound—"realize that the combination of tobacco amblyopia and the Capgras Syndrome, with the well-known character misidentification symptoms that Mrs. Collins vividly displays, adds up to vitamin-B12 deficiency or pernicious anemia, as already pointed out by the chief of neurology. The only problem, of course, is why doesn't Mrs. Collins have anemia?"

The audience was stilled by the hitherto unknown existence of the Capgras Syndrome and they feverishly wrote it down, along with the intriguingly named "*tobacco amblyopia*"—the latter, conjuring up the literary images painted in Erskine Caldwell's *Tobacco Road*, featuring scantily clad, long-limbed women with erotic urges.

"First described by the French psychiatrist Jean Marie Joseph Capgras, who observed that the patient's delusion was often that of a close friend or relative being replaced by an imposter, an exact double," I continued. "Hey, I'm sure you all remember the movie with the alien pods taking over the citizens of

Santa Mira. What the heck was that movie's name?" I asked, my head down as I eyed my notes in faux concentration.

"*The Invasion of the Body Snatchers*!" everyone shouted.

Audience participation was such a wondrous educational tool.

"Sometimes the sufferer thinks that their pet or even an inanimate object such as a sofa or book has been replaced by an exact replica. The patient is consciously aware of the changes, so it's not a hallucination."

"Thank you, Dr. Ted. Our senior student also discovered information for your edification," Dr. Zitfield moderated.

The student, well-coached, lectured with the authority of a more seasoned smart aleck. "As you all know, vitamin-B12 deficiency or pernicious anemia is masked by the administration of folic acid. One of Mrs. Collins's sons is a pharmacist, and we thought it possible that he provided her with a preparation containing that vitamin. Yesterday evening he confirmed that his mother does imbibe a potion of his own creation containing large amounts of folic acid. Folic acid treats the anemia, but not the neurologic abnormalities of B12 deficiency."

This student had potential. I'd ask the chief of medicine to interview him for residency training.

My turn again. I disliked giving up the floor.

"So we think Mrs. Collins has pernicious anemia as the cause of her neurological disease and her confusion. The cognoscenti know this as megaloblastic mania. It's manifested by tobacco amblyopia and the Capgras Syndrome, both of those disorders now old hat to you.

"The intra-muscular administration of 1000 micrograms of vitamin-B12 on a weekly basis for several months, and then monthly, should prompt complete improvement, perhaps even in as short a time as a few weeks. Please start it stat.

"Thank you all for the interesting consultation and for bearing with us for this long-winded explanation describing the infirmities affecting the lovely Mrs. Collins. We appreciate your confidence in us by asking our team to see and comment about her, and should there be any further questions, please don't hesitate to contact us at any time."

We humbly lowered our heads, gathered our papers, and quietly shuffled our way out of the conference room, victorious in our joust with the plebian neurologists. The slaughter rule was in effect. Not only had we provided a diagnosis for the neurologists, but it was a neurology diagnosis. And as a bonus, we helped Mrs. Collins, who, as predicted, morphed into her bright and normal self.

"Mrs. Collins, you look terrific," I offered at the follow-up examination just a month later during an unusual warm spell, the sun sprinkling through the windows and lighting up her face.

"Thank you, Doctor, and thanks for your help. It's okay, go ahead, light up a cigarette and blow smoke at me. Nothing bad will happen to my eyesight, but, of course, I'll have to report you to the hospital authorities for smoking." Showing off her wit, she laughed loud and hugged me close. All the good things we pray for.

# THREE

My good fortune, certainly not his, Stan Glicke was in the hospital and asking for me. Starting the antibiotics and making sure the infections didn't exacerbate his diabetes was my assignment.

Estelle, annoyance etched on her lovely face, walked out of his room, her index finger pointing toward me. "I'm not touching that man. He's loaded with gonorrhea and he only wants to see you. That figures, doesn't it Ted? A creep insisting on seeing only one doctor in the entire institution, and surprise, surprise, it's you."

I would have preferred to kiss her index finger, but instead I grabbed it, her mean words rushing my heart, while I repeated my oft-administered lecture to our colleagues who had abandoned Stan Glicke. "Remember, please, the Hippocratic Oath, the pledge we took when we graduated medical school—we help the sick, we succor the ill..." the latter followed by her great laugh.

"Good word, '*succor*,' I like that," she said. "You're a goddamn saint. Take care of your friend and maybe later I'll succor your ring, you big sucker." She laughed that great laugh of hers. But before abandoning Stan to me, Estelle added with concern, astute doctor that she was—"Ted, go look at Glicke's right knee. I'm worried about it. It's swollen and warm. I offered to aspirate it, but he wants you to look at it. *Only* you," she said, and with that she left, no touching, no hugs, no words of endearment, only the lingering fragrance of surgical scrub soap and spring flowers.

"Hey, *boychik*, good to see you—and that doctor who just left the room, what a honey." Stan greeted me with a grin in spite of his infirmities. "She nearly puked when she informed me the '*clap*' was in my throat and my nose.

"Ted, their combined ages were in the low double digits."Spoken wistfully—hospitalized and ill, and Glicke was still talking about tropical trysts. "And there were three or four of them—I kind of lost count. Life is good for those pure of heart."

Shaking my head in disgust, I asked my friend, "Didn't you take the antibiotics I gave you? Don't you ever think about healthy alternatives like miniature golf, or contract bridge, or God-forbid, even a meaningful relationship? One of these days, the infection will travel to your heart or brain and give you a stroke or a heart attack and make your diabetes go ballistic!"

"Ballistic! It was ballistic all right!" Stan gloated. "Better than a grand slam in a major with every finesse working, and you know, Ted, this was more fun than paying the bag ladies to sit on my nose and play bouncy. Hey, just kidding about that. I don't do weird things."

I aspirated Stan's knee. Swollen, angry-appearing, and bulging with fluid, Estelle, as usual, was right on the mark with her concerns. Stan handled the pain like a trooper, holding still, eyes closed, and taking long, deep breaths.

"Stan, thanks for suggesting I contact Sergeant Esposito. He's been helpful and he's a good guy." Stan needed distraction from the knee aspiration. I needed the talk.

"Listen carefully Ted. The sergeant isn't a good guy. He's a *goniff* like the rest of them. Don't trust him. But he knows everybody, and you asked me whom to contact about a homicide, right?"

Where had this negative version of George come from? So matter-of-fact now, and yet Stan had seemed so positive when he recommended I telephone the sergeant.

Leaving the needle in place, I told Stan to "hang loose, don't move," then I poured half of the joint fluid into a sterile culture tube and the remainder into a tube primed with heparin to prevent clotting for the white cell count and differential. Opening another syringe, I aspirated the remainder of the knee fluid. The thorough drainage would provide comfort.

"Stan, if I ever get into crime trouble," I asked, my mind functioning at several levels, my personal concerns rivaling his infections. "I can count on you to get me out of difficulty, can't I? I'm a physician and I provide patient care and avoid violence. And what do you mean George Esposito is like the rest of them?"

"Do you have any idea how many doctors I've represented over the years and all of them claiming to be descendents of Mohandas Gandhi?" Stan said, still lying still, but his brain fully charged. "Call me anytime. And, if you're ever questioned by the police about anything, the time of the day, your bowling handicap, your shoe size, don't trust them, say nothing. Give them my card," and with that, he reached over into the bedside table and handed me his embossed card as if all along he had been anticipating lawyer business. "Tell them you want to telephone me, stat. I don't care whether you're guilty or innocent, you're a good guy, especially if you get me better. By the way, not saying too much is good advice for all of life and here I'm giving it to you *gratis*. *Verstehen!*" Shrugging his shoulders, Stan assured me he was on my side: "now and forever." His words were similar to a wedding vow, and no further mention was made about my friend, the sergeant.

Neisseria infection, also known as "the clap," is difficult to culture from joint fluid under the best of circumstances. A fastidious organism, it dries out quickly outside the warm mucus membranes of the vagina, mouth, and urethra. You can't get gonorrhea from sitting on the toilet seat in spite of that wisdom provided to you by your phys-ed teacher and your best friends. When the attractive ladies tell me that's how they got the disease, I damn the filthy toilet seats right along with them, while I ponder whether to invite them to lunch.

I held the culture tube containing the knee fluid in the palm of my hand to keep it warm and hustled down to the microbiology laboratory. None of the technicians spoke English, and they also would ignore my instructions unless I stood there and watched them. "Place this fluid on a chocolate agar plate right now," I ordered.

I've screamed at them so often and in so many languages that they knew their path of least resistance was for them to just go-ahead and plate the joint fluid on the chocolate agar, the best media to grow the gonorrhea bugs. Its name, chocolate agar, described its color, the gelatinous culture media mixed with hemolyzed blood, the product taking on the appearance of Frango mints, but hardly its taste.

And all was well with Stan, the pain lessened, his mood brightened, the knee regained its shape, and we were on the right track. That was, until his fourth day of hospitalization when Stan's knee became trouble again—hot and swollen—just as it had been on his hospital admission.

"Doc, listen up, about my knee," Stan said. "If you're giving me the right antibiotic, why am I getting worse? Something's wrong here, isn't it? I dabble in malpractice law and the hospital has big pockets. Did you drool on the syringe and needle when you took out the knee fluid and now there's a new infection? My knee really hurts." Stan was pleading with me more than litigating, his hands out, seeking my help. The antibiotic he was receiving should have eradicated the Neisseria organism. The sensitivity testing performed in the laboratory had confirmed that.

I aspirated the knee fluid again. Surprised to find such cloudy fluid after several days of antibiotic treatment, I took a sample to the laboratory for another culture and for inspection under the microscope. No hassle from the sullen technicians, they had just finished breakfast in the cafeteria and Mrs. B had taken the starch out of them.

I commandeered their microscope and placed a drop of the fluid on a clean slide topped by a thin glass cover slip, and under high magnification view I found no bacteria bouncing around with Brownian movement—but in every field there were long, needle-shaped crystals clustered inside white blood cells.

Ken, the laboratory chief, suggested incubating a drop of the fluid with diluted uricase, the enzyme that digests gout crystals. We did, and it did: one drop of the diluted enzyme and the crystals disappeared as if by magic.

❖ ❖ ❖

"Stan, you have gout, no new infection," I told him, nearly knocking the door off his room in my excitement. "It's morning-report good news," I told him. "I'll start colchicine tablets, hopefully enough to relieve your knee pain and not enough to cause diarrhea." Colchicine was poison to the intestine, and running to the john was cumbersome, especially when burdened with a painful knee and intravenous lines attached to your arms.

"Ted, good news is good news, but you almost broke my door down. Thanks for the attention by the way, and even I know that gout is better than a new infection. Here's my gift for you, something I've thought about for a while. There's a girl in the islands who offers special meditation classes. Just the routine that would relax a high-energy guy like you—no sex, only conversation and music—it's designed for intellectuals like us. Sitting nearly naked on a rocking chair in the verandah with a mandolin on her lap, she plays any song you request. Broadway, classical, jazz, you name it. You rest your head on her legs—well actually, you bury your face high up on her soft thighs. Her skin feels young and warm on your cheeks and lips, and you slowly rock, back and forth, unwinding, your cares fading away faster than the chance of the White Sox winning the pennant." Stan talking wistfully, his eyes glazed over with fond remembrances.

"Stan what a wonderful talent and thanks for the vivid description," I said. "Let's schedule a recital for her at Symphony Hall with special pricing for front-row seats, but for now Stan, let's get over the gout and get you home."

# FOUR

Morning report had become repetitious, our only amusement was shouting at each other about trivial matters blown into life-and-death importance. How much potassium to add to the intravenous bottle, or which surgeons to avoid for intricate procedures? Today would be different, thanks to me and Stan Glicke.

The conference room was filled to capacity. There was a premonition about the events that were soon to unfold, my colleagues unusually alert as they jostled for prime seating. The doughnuts were long gone, and the tepid, dark coffee was on the verge of running out, while we lined up for refills milking the tall brown metal coffee containers tilted horizontal for the last tasteless drop. The stuff was free and when smothered with enough sugar and cream, provided a wake-up jolt.

The microscope borrowed from hematology had top-notch optics. I didn't trust our usual morning-report pizza-encrusted one for the fireworks I was preparing to display. This was going to be grand, like a Chicago Fourth of July celebration. *Big* like the *1812 Overture* played with real cannons broadcast over our paging system.

First came Stan's story of the knee pain, delivered without the carnal details of how he had contracted the infection. I described the results of Stan's first joint-fluid aspiration and solicited opinions regarding diagnoses. Information about the mandolin entertainer with the velvet thighs remained private. Who knew when I might need her services?

My colleagues correctly guessed the diagnosis. This was old hat to them. Stan had been admitted too many times before with his gonorrhea infections. We concurred about the selection of the appropriate antibiotic selection, and we posited that Stan would improve. And he did. So why, my associates asked, was I presenting this straightforward joint infection in this strange patient for discussion at morning report, our vehicle for education? Ennui settled in, eyelids drooped, and morning report became quieter than an IntMed picnic without Howard and me.

Time for Bombshell Number One!

"In spite of our brilliance and good intentions, and after initial improvement with the antibiotics, the patient worsened," I said. "His knee once again became painful, warm, and swollen. It was as if he had received no treatment at all." Pacing the floor with my dissertation, talking in sing-song fashion and pointing fingers, I recaptured the attention of my associates.

"What are we doing wrong?" I asked. "How have we failed this upstanding citizen of our fair city, who entrusted his medical care and life to our esteemed teaching hospital and the golden hands and sophisticated minds present in all of you?

"Tell me, tell me, tell me now, what should we do?" The alliteration and euphony were extracted from long ago bedtimes shared with Dr. Seuss.

"Right!" I said after the pregnant pause. "No one has a clue as to what's going on. But I do, and in my graciousness, I'll share it with you. Educating the common man and woman, the 'little people' so to speak, high school graduates all to be sure, is one of my missions in life.

"Everyone, please line up in an orderly fashion, single file, women first, and gander into the microscope I have readied for you. Placed there is a drop of the patient's joint fluid I aspirated yesterday, when the knee was swelling and the pain recurred with a vengeance. If you're observant, and if your thinking caps are in place, you'll discover great wisdom, because the diagnosis will be apparent, right in front of your eyes to even the slowest among you."

After my associates saw the crystals lying inside the white blood cells, I would add a drop of the uricase solution to the slide, and to their amazement the crystals would dissolve, establishing the diagnosis of gout and the cause of Stan's pain. Sitting on top of the world with my medical magic, I was beginning to hear appreciative murmurs from my colleagues as they peered into the microscope.

Then Bombshell Number Two!

Mrs. Gail burst in the room—no knocking, no apologies to the chief for the trespass, her high-heeled *clomps* synchronized with the squeak of the front door flinging back and forth. Her customary smirk was replaced by concern, contorting her mouth downward, and understandably so, because crowding and dwarfing her were Sergeant George Esposito and two bulky uniformed policemen.

George dismissed Mrs. Gail with a curt nod of his head, and walked toward the chief. The city's finest, big and beefy, made their way to the two doors, arms akimbo, facing the young doctors, blocking the exits, enjoying their authority, saddened only by the absence of frosted doughnuts and long johns.

George talked to the chief, *sotto voce,* while he searched the room, one doctor after another, until finding me.

"I have a search warrant for the apartment of Dr. Tadeusz Shluzkinski and an arrest warrant for the same doctor regarding the death of a Mr. Tim Schmidt," he said, waving a very official-appearing document. "If the doctor is in the room, please step forward." He was playing the crowd for all it was worth, knowing full well where I was.

All eyes centered on me as I spoke over the otherworldly quiet. "George, it's so good to see you so early in the morning and so unexpectedly." My voice was strong. "Would you be kind enough to allow me one moment, please, while I place a drop of this important enzyme on this microscope slide?" And I did, not waiting for his reply.

"Everybody," I said, speaking to my associates, "please form a line at the microscope just as you so capably did before. Sergeant, you and your friends are welcome to join in. But be orderly now," I cautioned. "Come on, folks, no pushing or shoving.

"Please notice the dissolution of the previously observed crystals with the addition of uricase." I lifted the bottle of enzyme over my head, gently waving it back and forth like the languid dance of a Calcutta cobra under the spell of a snake charmer's *pungi.* "It proves beyond doubt, even amongst those of you less gifted in problem-solving, that the crystals you observed just moments ago in the joint fluid of our patient are sodium urate crystals.

"Thus," I continued, "I think it reasonable to assume that our patient's new problem is gout. A reasonable assumption, being that the gout crystals were already present in the joint, innocently residing there, never causing trouble, so to speak, until being washed out from their hiding places by inflammation caused by the gonorrhea infection. *Debrided*, I believe, is the more sophisticated term to describe that event. Gout, of course, is easily treatable.

"Thank you all for allowing me to weave together this fascinating and instructive story on this early morning. I'm sure it's piqued your interest. A follow-up discussion about the patient's course will be provided at a time to be announced later," I said, spoken as my gendarme friend and old confidant handcuffed me with thick, shiny metal cuffs previously doubled up on his belt and now jangling louder than the bells on Santa's sleigh leading the annual State Street Christmas Parade. My arms were shackled in front and not behind me, which I assumed was a courtesy based on our previous friendship.

This episode, sure to live on in morning report legend, was a first for the chief, Mrs. Gail, and the entire Department of Medicine. And it was especially intriguing for my colleagues, who were unsure whether this was Act One of a comedy routine conjured up by me and my best friend and coconspirator, Howard, or the real thing.

I remembered not to say anything to Sergeant Esposito.

# FIVE

Picture yourself in a bustling institution where doctors were kings, and in deference to the many ill patients, silence was strictly enforced. Tack a tumultuous parade onto those tenets, the walk of the condemned, for instance, and a doctor no less. Think the Bataan death march in double time; or maybe the Ringling Brothers Circus high-stepping down Main Street on opening day, with somersaulting clowns and dancing acrobats winding their way through the hospital corridors heading toward the entrance, brightly attired, several in police uniforms, others in white coats, bunched together and with dozens of newcomers randomly popping in and out.

Imagine the finale of Tchaikovsky's *Peter and the Wolf*, the grandfather portrayed by the chief, who shook his head in bewilderment, the policemen taking the roles of the hunters, violins serenading the hospital workers and visitors with Peter's melody. The captured wolf, head held high, still proud, in handcuffs, being played by yours truly, wearing a white coat for this performance, his stethoscope knocked ajar from the jostling and dangling down from his left-hand side pocket, earpieces scraping the floor. Two gendarmes on either side, stern and expressionless, but just beneath the surface, if you looked carefully you could note a whiff of levity.

"*Take him to the zoo, the zoo, we've captured him alive*" cried Peter, played by Sergeant Esposito, but for this performance only, the words were, "Take him to jail."

Mrs. Gail, the trusty bird companion, clip clopping by my side, asked endearingly, how she could help? Howard and I exchanged glances, another adventure unfolding. Mrs. B, openmouthed, her fantasies about my downfall less striking than this fascinating parade marching right in front of her. Jane, lovely Jane, asked to see the sergeant's arrest warrant and who could refuse her, my friend and the hospital lawyer who whispered in my ear, "Don't say anything." It was the lawyer's mantra.

What was the chief thinking, while caught up in this unwanted event? Would he run out of pipe tobacco and Scotch today?

Past the gift shop, the elevators, the admission office, the cashier, the information desk, and the lobby, the hospital hushed as if it was 1 a.m. on a night before a national holiday. Estelle, Sophie, Amy, Mother and Harry, thanks for not being here at the time of my humiliation.

The cold air rushed my face as the automatic door swished open, the wind storming off the lake, adding realism to the surrealistic quality of the march of the doomed. My head was protected by a policeman's hand inserted between the roof and my scalp, while I was being pushed into the backseat of the squad car—exactly the way it's depicted in the movies. The roof lights revolved; the headlights flashed on and off automatically. I expected the clowns to join us, but the car doors snapped shut with a resounding *click* of the locks, sealing me in.

George turned around from the front passenger seat of the patrol car and loosened my handcuffs. "Friend, don't do anything silly," he told me. I nodded acquiescence. My three captors started laughing.

"Doc," the uniformed driver spoke. "I hope you're innocent of whatever we're taking you in for, but speaking for myself, that was the best arrest I ever made. Did you ever see so many open mouths and dancing feet? Wait until I tell the girls at Maddie's about this escapade. If that doesn't get me laid, I don't know what will. Sergeant, we should have had a photographer, we and the doctor here would be famous."

These were my kind of people as I watched them laugh. Three out of four of us enjoyed the mirth of the fun handcuffing and the high-stepping antics.

George outlined the morning's activity while we drove north. "Ted, we'll search your apartment. Your help, of course, will be welcomed. If we find your handgun, we'll bring you to the station and hold you until ballistics are performed. And, my friend, if we don't find the weapon, like it's suddenly been stolen or misplaced or something on that bullshit order, we'll have to book you for possible murder—and speaking for myself, Doc, that will be very disappointing. It's what we call in police parlance, a lose-lose situation. Sorry about that, my friend."

I would have preferred silence, but cops like to talk. George, after being cooped up at his desk all day, relished conversation with a perpetrator. That was what he'd suffered through police school for.

"We ran the list of guns purchased recently, guns like the one that wasted Tim Schmidt," he droned, "and lo and behold, your name popped up. I told my boss it must be a mistake, that you wouldn't be so careless or plain dumb. But as you can see, we're here with the warrants. It would be a feather in the captain's cap to solve the murder of a mob chieftain, especially with the wonderful publicity surrounding the arrest of a physician from a prestigious institution. Too bad there isn't a young and beautiful woman involved and/or a serial killer—but there isn't and you're not one, are you, my friend?"

Glad we were still performing vaudeville. I just smiled, not talking to the police, following Stan's and Jane's cogent instructions.

Well-marked police cars with blinking flashers have the luxury of speeding down crowded streets and not struggling to find parking spaces, spoiling the civilian time of the drivers as they chauffeur the family to the convenience store for milk and cigarettes and need to fend off the rest of the pushy populace for coveted parking slots.

The driver and my backseat companion exited first, directly in front of my apartment house, flush in between the no parking signs, shifting their belts upward with their panoply of goodies, revolvers, radios, flashlights, handcuffs, and nightsticks, with well-practiced body wiggles. George helped me exit, one hand firmly around my biceps, the other keeping my head safe.

Midmorning and the street was busy, passersby intrigued by our posse. Me in my doctor's uniform, stethoscope still dangling near my feet, the four of us possibly comprising a new type of strike force, maybe the anti-germ warfare-squad, an excellent after dinner conversation topic for the kids and spouse. Mrs. Linderman, my next-door neighbor and protector, who was just leaving the building for her morning chores, the cleaners, the post office, the grocery store, said hello to us with her generous smile, unaware in her gentler view of the world that anything might be amiss.

"Ted, tell you friends"—acknowledging all of us with a sweeping hand—"that Kroger's is having a two-for-one sale on soft drinks. Coca-Cola is included, not their house-brand trash. Have you ever in God's name tasted their so-called root beer? It's real *root,* all right, rooted in Blandsville," she said, followed by a guffaw. "Can I pick up something for you? Should I see if they're discounting real beer?"

Mrs. Linderman and I frequently enjoyed a cold Hamm's while solving some of the world's problems. Before closing up shop, we would toast Mr. Linderman, the beer bottles empty except for one last swig, as we honored the beloved veteran of WWII, long-interred in the cemetery near the VA hospital in the western suburbs.

The four of us thanked Mrs. Linderman, the two uniformed policemen graciously removing their caps because no one was in a hurry and the day was young and I didn't pose much of a threat. Who knew when they might need a medical opinion about their rash or cough or that funny-looking thing growing on their member?

Two by two, we walked up the one flight of stairs to my apartment. And just before I fished the keys out of my worn slacks, a difficult task with manacled hands, and handed them to my detective friend, he turned to me with seriousness written on his face, and told me there was something he needed to say. Something he had thought about at great length. "Ted, my doctor buddy, take this suggestion from a guy who has seen shit from every angle. Retribution has its own course. It can't be hurried, and it doesn't belong to us." Maybe this counsel was something I should have taken seriously, although it was a bit late for it now.

"Thanks for the sage advice, George," I told him. It was given to me as a friend, while we entered my musty, not-so-bachelor-like apartment, thanks to Sophie's goading, cleaning, and straightening.

"Gentlemen," I implored, "please accompany me while I go to my closet and retrieve something that should make your stay here a short one."

The four of us squeezed amoeba-like through my bedroom door, sliding by my desk, chair neatly in place, reading material piled symmetrically and orderly, in-box filled with medical journals, out-box piled with fiction and girlie magazines. The closet door stuck shut as always, not always the carpenter's fault, these old buildings settle even in our seismically quiet city, but it finally opened with a thud.

You can take the measure of a man by the state of his garage or workbench or closet. I failed. The smell of the Keds and stale sweat clothes from my more athletic aspirations, piled up randomly, and taking all the closet space, momentarily choked us, the familiarity of the stench not affording me a modicum of immunity.

I awkwardly reached overhead to locate my pistol on the upper shelf, above the shirts and slacks on hangers. No artificial patting around the closet shelf, no fake attestations of, "*I know it was here just a day or so ago, where can it be*?" This was serious. No games.

I handed the box to George.

And it was pristine. Identical to the day when I brought it home from Big Al's. The .45-caliber handgun, neatly encased in its form-fitting cardboard packing covered with cellophane was unchanged from the day I purchased it. The gleaming metal, brand new, never fired, no scratches around the barrel tip for a silencer, the untouched, unsullied, virgin package provided my alibi. It screamed to the world: "*Free this innocent doctor, this gun was never even unwrapped.*"

Howard and I made copies of our favorite cartoon ripped from a *New Yorker* magazine. It pictured a circus trainer shaking his downcast head while sitting next to his recently deceased elephant lying motionless on its side in the center of the main circus ring. The handler, speaking aloud, but to no one in particular said: "Some days nothing seems to go right." My day was the antithesis. Tension dissipated as quickly as the ride to my apartment. Lady Luck and good fortune arrived together, hand in hand, blue skies appeared overhead, the air fresh and spring-like, thoroughly displacing the penetrating odor of fear that had enveloped me just minutes ago.

Sergeant George Esposito was on the phone with his captain. "This .45 has the correct ID number, but it's never been used. It's still securely wrapped from the manufacturer," George said, his voice lowering, his hand over the speaker, "and the barrel has never been tampered with."

George beckoned to me, still on the phone, one hand placed over the mouthpiece. "Doc, you're free to go back to work. Don't leave town, and your armament, it goes to the crime lab to be sure it's really as pristine as it looks." He fussed with the key to remove my handcuffs, barely paying attention to me. I had become a lousy innocent. My unmanacled wrists felt wonderful. The absence of pain brings pleasure.

George turned away to more police business, likely discussing vacation plans, finally hanging up, barked orders to his minions, gave a pat on the back for me, and then he departed. The door was left wide open. No apologies. No receipt for the pistol. No offer to drive me anywhere. My car was at the hospital.

Noontime and I was exhausted. The physical and mental fatigue of being dragged through the hospital was the equivalent of being on call two nights in a row. It was more exhausting than a day spent assisting a cranky surgeon performing a Whipple procedure going sour.

Jane was on the telephone, good lawyer that she was, telling me once more to keep quiet. She would meet me at the police station. "Jane, the police have already left, my arrest was a mistake. There are no charges or anything against me that I'm aware of, and I'm planning to return to work. Would you kindly inform the chief and Mrs. Gail about this change in events, and I'll explain to them what happened this morning when I return."

I was going to ask Stan Glicke what we could do about countering the humiliation of my morning's walk through the hospital. However, I knew that by tomorrow, if not sooner, my status in the medical community would attain its zenith, as valuable to my notoriety as being the first author of a lead article in the *New England Journal of Medicine*, our most prestigious journal. It would be similar to being a former NFL player or movie star in the residency program, the only downside being the continuous stares from the younger doctors and students and the fallout of having all medical decisions closely scrutinized.

Maybe I'm exaggerating—maybe being cuffed and led out of my own hospital by the police wouldn't enhance my reputation, but I still needed to hold my head high.

I showered—the second of the day, washing off the anxiety—found fresh clothes and cabbed back to the hospital. Mrs. Gail said to go right in, added respect in her eyes for my recent brush with fame. After all, how many potential felons could she boss around? On the other hand, her kindness was being fiercely tested by the morning's activities, which were disrupting any constructive plans she had scheduled.

The chief listened and good listener that he was, made my explanation easier, although, not necessarily truthful. I told him about Tim's murder and my previous meeting with Sergeant Esposito, in which I'd discussed my concerns about Betty's fate with him.

"I purchased a gun after my beating that was similar to the one used to kill Tim Schmidt," I told the chief. "It was a mistake purchasing a handgun. I know that now, but I was angry. I'm not used to being on the wrong side of a physical altercation, especially one so devastating. The weapon was never used and remained stored away, sealed in the box it came in." Then I paused before speaking again. "And I'm embarrassed about the purchase."

My lies were coming easy as I continued. "The police are looking at the pistol, but it's never been fired." A lot of true, true statements, but not necessarily related, similar to the written examinations we were subjected to throughout medical school. The chief didn't offer sympathy. Going to the police as I did when Betty died and owning a handgun were acts outside of his purview of correctness. He looked closely at me, trying to make sense of my thoughts, my different background, my motives, until, with the slightest nod of his head, he decided in my favor.

"Of course you're innocent. You're an excellent and caring doctor. You wouldn't think about committing murder. But, Ted, I worry about you. Some students don't live up to their potential because of poor work habits or lack of commitment or having no common sense or just not enough brain power. Those are certainly not your problems, but for some reason you don't fit into the mainstream of doctors who train here. You're smart and, believe it or not, I like your sense of humor. But you're always battling authority and having difficulty controlling your impulses, and that's limiting your success.

"Ted, this morning's show with the diagnosis of gout in the patient with multiple sites of infection should have permanently enhanced your reputation. But who's going to remember that stellar, magician like presentation after an arrest warrant delivered in person by one of our city's finest and you subjected to being handcuffed in morning report and paraded through the hospital? Everywhere I went this morning, they were talking about it—not how much insulin to administer to the diabetic patient, or how to titrate digitalis in the congestive heart failure sufferer—it was about Dr. Ted being arrested in morning report! Believe me, Ted, I've thought about you a lot. Go back to work, but first telephone Dr. Edith Gershon in Psychiatry and schedule an appointment to see her. She's expecting your call."

# SIX

Tall, with dark hair, a sturdy and forceful gait, and a disarming smile, Dr. Gershon's counsel could offset evil thoughts. The psychiatry-medicine liaison team she had organized was busier than the newborn nursery. Many of our patients and even more of our students and medical residents at some time during their training needed guidance, or drugs, or hospitalization for their emotional scars, personality disorders, and the pressure of working sixty to seventy hours per week.

We met on the tennis court early in my first year. Dr. Gershon, proud of her tennis expertise, needed to embarrass the young men foolish enough to take the game lightly. I played the game as if we were at center court Wimbledon, or as if it were a boxing match combined with an overlay of rugby with money wagered on the outcome. I would smash the ball at her or at her feet and savor the winning shot—she was a psychiatrist, after all, and more than capable of handling adversity. And I provided her with a workout, plus, of course, it was therapy for me. In medical circles that's called a "twofer."

Today, we discussed my "in your face" behavior and let bygones be bygones from our tennis endeavors. And, of course, there was my purchase of a handgun, an unheard-of act in our profession, the dreams of my beating by the two thugs, the deaths of patients including Betty, and the shouting matches with hospital personnel—I was a cornucopia of pathology, a potential lifetime project.

"Ted," she wisely told me at the beginning of our first session, "when you're ready to boil over, stop what you're doing. Completely stop. Sit down, even rest your chin on your chest and ask yourself, *Why do I feel so shitty and irritable? Did I get enough sleep? Have I missed a meal? Did I forget to say I care for someone important*?" There was no badinage. "Those are the things you need to think about before becoming angry or irrational or performing acts that you'll regret later. Remember this message. Take it to heart."

"Maybe as I get older, I'll quiet down, at least a little, but I hear what you're saying and thank you," I said.

We discussed my relationships with women, my fantasies about Estelle, my concerns about Sophie, and my constant battles with women in authority, Mrs. B and Mrs. Gail high up on my list, not mentioning Dr. Gershon herself. My childhood was talked about and in detail, and we agreed there existed a surfeit of love at all times, allowing a solid emotional base for us to work with.

# SEVEN

Thank you, Sophie. Women were the true God, a morning rendezvous, an afternoon coffee, and I quick-stepped through the rest of the day.

Dr. Mollman called. It's unusual for his highness to personally telephone an applicant. He offered me the job in Dr. Brennan's laboratory and first crack at a clinical fellowship for the following year. His exact words were: "Unless you screw up, there will be a position available." Since I screw up a lot, his offer didn't necessarily reassure me.

I asked him—"please"—yes, I really used the word *please*, to place the offer in writing and include the financial arrangements so that I could show it to Jane. Dr. Mollman had expected me to bless him for his papal-like offering, not ask about compensation or to have anything placed in writing and reviewed by a lawyer, but he acquiesced, and I promised him my best effort. Floating in air, my feet barely touching the floor, Fred Astaire in *Flying Down to Rio* I danced the carioca down the corridors to tell Herb Rhoban, the chief, Howard, and Sophie, the news.

❖ ❖ ❖

My next two weeks were spent on the General Medicine Service—my last rotation on the busy admission and inpatient service, two more weeks of servitude, time that my comrades weren't subjected to, but thanks to Mrs. Gail, I had the special opportunity to lose sleep and expend energy. Every third day and night, my team admitted and initiated treatment for all of the hospital medical admissions. That's when I met Mr. Ray.

He came rolling in late one night, express from the nursing home, confused, lethargic, febrile, coughing, and short of breath.

"What came first, sir, the sputum or the shortness of breath?" I yelled at him in the overcrowded emergency room, while I prodded him with my stethoscope and reflex hammer. Seeing me dressed in my white coat, Mr. Ray crossed himself and clammed up, assuming I was his personal angel of death. He'd be damned if he was going to smooth his way to a higher place. We were forced to treat him with digitalis and diuretics for congestive heart failure and antibiotics for pneumonia.

During my early work rounds the next morning, while the world still shaded dark, I had time to digest the laboratory and X-ray results and sit down with our charges—that was when I recognized Mr. Ray. He was the radio ventriloquist, the entertainer, whose lips moved when the dummy spoke, his skills the antithesis of "throwing" one's voice in spite of the illustrated instructions in his popular booklet on how to become a famous ventriloquist in five easy lessons for 25 cents and two Wheaties box tops (*please no postage stamps*). Clever on the radio, but on late-afternoon children's television, Mr. Ray's lack of skill became apparent even to adolescents such as me. Before each broadcast, the studio audience was sternly cautioned to refrain from pointing and shouting: "He's moving his lips!"

And, of course, there was Donnie, the wise-cracking doll, handsomely dressed in tuxedo and bow tie, sitting primly on Mr. Ray's lap, turning on his benefactor at every opportunity and challenging him to be a "real" ventriloquist.

Donnie was joined by Mr. Ray's lovely assistant, Annemarie, the beauty with the acerbic tongue. Dressed in high-riding skirts and low-slung blouses exposing gorgeous flesh, she would lean over Donnie while singing the popular songs of the day that were the mainstay of the show. While caressing the doll, Annemarie would stare at me, as I watched the show on our first-on-the block, black-and-white twelve-inch, General Electric television set.

Senior medical residents such as I, tired of performing minor procedures or writing orders or partaking in routine decision-making—after all we knew everything there was to know—promoted our students and first-year residents for those chores. Sitting with our feet up, we supervised the day-to-day activities from afar, only participating with the fun stuff—the spinal punctures, the pericenteses, the thoracenteses, except for Mr. Ray. He was my baby. No one was permitted to touch him, while I shepherded him through recovery.

Pulling strings, I arranged for his transfer to our rehabilitation unit, no nursing home return for him. I snuck into his room at his old-age palace, grabbed the Donnie doll, oiled it up, and prodded the hospital's audio and visual service to provide the sixteen-millimeter camera and film. The surgery scrub technician removed Mr. Ray's facial stubble with a straight razor; I gave him a fresh, long sleeved shirt purchased from the hospital gift shop, buttoned it up to the neck, and we were set to go. The last Mr. Ray show. And he was eager enough to be the real Mr. Ray, the radio ventriloquist, just as he had been on television years ago.

Howard played the piano and sang. Jane, now known as Annemarie, danced with Donnie, Sophie was Patsy Klein, the almost-famous country singer, and I directed this long absent urbanity for posterity.

Mr. Ray said, "Let's sing that new ballad together—*Vaya con Dios*— please Donnie, Annemarie and Patsy, a one, a two..."

Donnie not singing, "Is that song Spanish, Mr. Ray?"

"Like a mazurka, gavotte or waltz, it's Spanish, all right," Mr. Ray answered.

"Will my Spanish princess Ava Gardner come by and sing it with me?" asked Donnie.

"Miss Gardner isn't Spanish, Donnie. You must be thinking of Sophia Loren," Mr. Ray responded.

Donnie, his voice identical to Mr. Ray's, spoke to the camera with his trade mark cheekiness, wooden arms flapping up and down like a windup wooden parrot. "Mr. Ray, I don't sing Spanish. If English is good enough for Marcel Marceau, it should be good enough for everyone. Why, just yesterday, I was strolling down Cermak Road and Wentworth Avenue, and all the speech I heard was foreign garble, clatter, and more clatter— why I thought ..."

Annemarie and Mr. Ray yelling in unison, "Donnie, for goodness sake, you were in Chinatown!"

Then there were the famous guests who canceled their appearance on the show at the last moment with fateful telephone calls taken live on television by

Mr. Ray, who was unable to mask his disappointment. Except for Patsy Klein, who had settled in as a regular. The country singer with the Yiddish sayings, she'd sing to Mr. Ray with her trademark clarity and trill: "I'll sing *bubkes* on this show unless there is cash in my envelope and not newspaper shreds like last time, you *goniff*."

The pièce de résistance was Donnie and Annemarie insisting that Mr. Ray drink from a glass of water while talking for Donnie, just like a real ventriloquist would. "It's unseemly and uncalled for," Mr. Ray would say, look resignedly at the audience, pause for several beats that seemed to last for an eternity, then swallow the water, and at the same time release a Dictaphone tape hidden inside the doll so it appeared that Donnie was speaking after all. It was amazing.

Mr. Ray would then lean forward and start choking, as if to cough-up the water, but the water would shoot out of Donnie's mouth from an enema syringe also hidden inside the doll. We would howl. Mr. Ray would beam.

There were sparks in Mr. Ray's eyes as he relived his show. Facial wrinkles and frown lines vanished while he graciously accepted accolades for the first time in more than a decade amid joyful memories for Howard, Jane, Sophie, and me that we had filmed for posterity.

On the following Monday, Mrs. Gail phoned. "The pleasure of your company is expected at five p.m."

Was I pleased! Such an endearing way of summoning me: the "pleasure of my company—indeed. But she did disconnect abruptly and didn't request a RSVP. For sure, the chief must be congratulating me about my new position at the university. A glass of his Scotch, feet up on the desk, two good old docs talking about research opportunities, life in the fast lane, discussing which laboratories were making progress and which ones were living on past reputations. You worked hard, traveled the straight and narrow, and good things happened.

Dr. Gershon had heard about our Mr. Ray show. Few secrets remain buried in hospitals. "Do you remember the episode when Lonnie, Donnie's twin, the puppet stricken with polio, was burnt to a crisp?" she asked. "Toast, they called him when his cardboard iron lung caught fire." The unfortunate result of a shamefully neglected bare electric wire, the tragedy captured live on television—the infamous "cardboard iron lung tragedy." Funny, how something so tragic can boost ratings. The funeral procession featured the entire Mr. Ray cast, strutting around the stage, singing the popular song "*Auf Wiedersehen*" for the beloved Lonnie.

Dr. Gershon and I sang the solemn words together and recalled the burial "at sea" as Lonnie's ashes were flushed down the women's staff toilet located just behind the center stage. The bulky old television camera crashing into the narrow doorway walls recording the event.

Mrs. Gail glanced up when I arrived, gracefully nodding her head toward the chief's office. Apparently, I could just walk in. I blew her a kiss.

"Ted, my interesting friend," the chief said, shaking his noble head after I took my usual seat. "I heard about the abuse showered on the ill Mr. Ray. I've already talked to Howard and Jane about the debacle. You orchestrated a ventriloquism show here at our hospital! Mr. Ray told his children that he might be leaving the nursing home and going on tour. What must I do with you? The time spent with Dr. Gershon in Psychiatry, what happened to that? Where are the results? When are the good decisions coming?"

He opened the desk drawer, not reaching for the bottle of Scotch, but rather for his pipe, packing it just right, lighter blazing, *puff, puff*, until he was ready for me. This was another first for him, a ventriloquism act in his hospital, masterminded by his senior resident and troublemaker, *puff, puff*, his mind presumably cranking out punishments.

"His children are very upset. *Very upset,* to put it mildly." The chief paused with his puffing. "They informed me that getting Mr. Ray to even agree to enter the nursing home took a great deal of persuasion. And rumor has it that now Mr. Ray and some yet-to-be identified medical resident have scheduled a sing-along in the Rehabilitation Unit, featuring the song from *Moulin Rouge* where the singers dance on their knees, as if they're midgets.

"Where is the professionalism?

"This takes the cake."

I tried to stifle my laughter, but I couldn't, laughing through my fingers spread horizontal over my mouth, and it became contagious, spreading fast across the desk like the Spanish flu.

I had never seen the chief laugh out loud before. Mrs. Gail, peeking in from outside the office door also laughed and pointed to the chief, as she apparently had never seen him laugh before either.

"What does Mr. Ray have to do with your platelet research next year with Drs. Brennan and Mollman?" the chief blurted. "I loved Mr. Ray," the chief continued. "I watched it with my children, and I remember the show where the entire cast danced on their knees to that song from *Moulin Rouge*, you know from the movie about Toulouse-Lautrec. Their guest star had to be rolled off the stage; he couldn't walk for weeks with his swollen knees. *Thud, thud, thud*, his knees keeping time with the music, oh my, that brings back so many memories."

"Do you two remember the show when Mr. Lawrence Welk telephoned and told Mr. Ray that he wasn't going to appear on the show after all?" Mrs. Gail said, pointing to us, her face aglow with happy memories. "He thought the invitation was for the *Hit Parade,* or the *Edgar Bergen and Charlie McCarthy Show.* Poor Mr. Ray tried to hide his disappointment, mouth quivering, but he recovered nicely, trooper that he was. Edging past the line of women waiting to pee, Mr. Ray ignored their mean-spirited comments, grabbed the liquid soap container from the sink, placed the solution in his water glass, extracted a wand from Donnie's suitcase, and started blowing bubbles, the way children do on a sunny summer afternoon while frolicking on the back porch. Mr. Ray smiled sweetly at the audience and danced around, a step here, a step there, pleased with himself, pleased with his very own Lawrence Welk bubble machine. And there were plenty of bubbles."

"Then Mr. Ray, anointed the three of them: Annemarie, Patsy and Donnie," I said, my turn to contribute to the circus, "the latter outfitted with a swirling skirt and a crimson wig snatched from Raggedy Ann, to play the Lennon Sisters.

"What'll you going to sing for the folksa, girls?' were Mr. Ray's exact words."

"And what song did they sing, Doctor?" Little Mrs. Gail pointed at me, testing my memory, index finger in the familiar accusatory position, challenging me, but with a grin spreading across her face.

I returned the smile, just as sweet, perhaps even more so, and speaking for the ersatz Lennon Sisters answered "Well, Mr. Ray, we're going to sing a favorite for all the folksa in television land, a one and a two"—and I started singing and boldly reached for Mrs. Gail's hand and sang a Johnny Mathis song: "*You turn to me with a kiss in your eyes...*"

Mrs. Gail stopped, regaining her senses, a combination of hand-holding and the mention of a kiss, the spell carried too far, as she stepped back from Johnny Mathis and me.

Out came the Scotch, a drizzle for me in a paper cup, full shot-glasses for the chief and Mrs. Gail. The chief, seeing my expression at his penurious offering, banged the table, glanced at Mrs. Gail and pointed to my crestfallen expression, then reached into his desk drawer and brought out a real glass for me. Scotch never tasted so good.

# EIGHT

Maria Amoroso wanted to speak to me about Tim Schmidt. Hard at work, she was sorting out early evening medicines in the small drug room set off from the nurses' station on 3GM, neatly recording each transaction in the daily ledger. She ladled the tablets and liquids into the fringed white paper medicine cups, smiled, and talked to me without missing a beat.

"Dr. Ted, when I was home in the Philippines, I thought about Betty Schmidt, you know the patient with lupus. I thought about what I told you. Sometimes my English isn't so good"—now she looked at me, interrupting her work for a moment—you're such a good doctor, Dr. Ted. Maybe I could teach you Tagalog—*magandang araw!*—that means a 'beautiful day' or 'good morning.' I'll take you home with me and have you meet my family. My two children stay with their father and their grandmothers. I'm their main support."

"I didn't realize you had a family," I said. Of course I didn't realize it. I never asked Maria about her personal life, social clod that I was, in spite of her kind words.

"Dr. Ted, do you remember when you asked me whether Betty's husband, I think his name was Tim, was in the room with his wife the night she died? I thought a lot about that night, but you know I'm still not sure if I remember it correctly. Sometimes things cloud my memory, especially with the pace so hectic around here. But I said yes to you that Tim, the husband, was heading toward the elevator. Now I think that Tim left a long time before, maybe just when I started my shift."

I internalized the jolt.

Maria paused to search her memory, her eyes still resting on me. "Later in the evening the engineer came to the floor to help repair the call lights in the next room and at the nurses' station, you know Jim the engineer. I think I mixed up my words, *Tim* with *Jim*. I meant to say that Jim was around Betty's room."

"Oh, no, Dr. Ted," Maria was adamant, "no one would pressure me about saying this. I just wanted to make sure you knew better what I said to you. And I traveled back home to the Philippines because it was vacation time. No one came to visit me here."

Maria was absolute about her recollection. My goodbye to her, "*ba-bay*," the extent of my Tagalog, was barely audible and slow.

Why did George say that Maria had been visited by Tim's goons?

Would I have to apologize to Tim in the afterlife?

But then if Tim suffocated Betty, he wouldn't have waited around.

I had no one to talk to about this change in perspective. The good Lord hadn't corresponded with me lately. Maybe speaking to Howard would fill the void.

Murder was such a lonely profession.

# NINE

Morning report was another tedious presentation about a hyperglycemic, ketotic diabetic patient, not taking adequate insulin, imbibing too much alcohol, and found in a coma. Our doctors, as usual, administered too much insulin and not enough fluids. The conversation stopped, awaiting my disparaging comments, but I just offered a thin smile. There were too many items crowding my mind, especially regarding Sophie.

Our intimacy was waning. I went far out of my way to be gracious, which was no great selling point. But I tried. As requested, I fashioned a Sunday morning breakfast in bed, only missing the Johnnie Ray music she requested. The record was warped from its pivotal role in our ersatz Frisbee game, but I babbled the pretty words of "Please, Mr. Sun."

Frozen waffles with artificial maple syrup and crispy bacon were artfully lined up around the edges of the scalloped paper plate as large as a full moon. The concoction was embellished by a glob of dairy fresh butter smack-dab in the center, perfectly mimicking a saffron-colored midsummer Shasta daisy.

Sophie knew how much I detested breakfast in bed. It was as overrated as making love on the couch or reading in the bathtub what with the scattered crumbs, the bunched-up sitting positions like lowercase *hs*, the getting up and down for forgotten items, and the syrup cementing our fingers together firmer than Elmer's Paste. But Elmer's was a delicacy compared with the outdated sugar syrup, and the frozen waffles' edges that were tougher than leather—the coffee was barely tepid, and when spilled in the middle of the bed it left a stain difficult to explain. Was there anything quite like breakfast in bed to dampen the promise of romance?

Sophie consented to come over for dinner in spite of the PB&J and cream cheese punishment and last week's breakfast in bed. The side dish of potato chips added the right contrast. Pretzels work just as well. It's the salt that complements the peanut butter. I know these culinary facts. I could author a book about gourmet dining, and maybe I will after years of preparing quick and nutritious dinners as a medical school and medical resident bachelor: *101 Quick and Easy Ways to Prepare Satisfying and Nutritious Dinners with Nabisco Wheat Squares Plus or Minus Kraft's Velveeta Cheese*, next on my creative agenda.

We worked off the calories, on top, on the bottom, on our sides, hands stroking here and there, and just before our passion and before Sophie moved up on my chest, I felt the skin lesions dotting her legs. Sophie had multiple punctate lesions on her thighs. Each one angry and red, the centers were pinpointed with black crust, indicating the presence of necrosis.

"I've been referred to the university for a rheumatology consultation," she said. Her words and the mean-looking sores were capably functioning as an anti-aphrodisiac. "The health service doctor was concerned about the possibility of vasculitis," Sophie continued.

I didn't think so. Sophie was otherwise well and without fever. It didn't seem right. Vasculitis was fatigue, weight loss, and fever, and all sorts of other bad things. It was only Sophie's mood that was shit. She shook her head when I offered to accompany her to the appointment.

A week later and Sophie read the skin biopsy results to me. "The intensity of the inflammation surrounding the blood vessels, although only modest, is most suggestive of the presence of vasculitis."

The doctors suggested a trial of prednisone.

Prednisone, the life-saving medicine that Betty Schmidt had taken was associated with a myriad of terrible side effects: weight gain, hypertension, insomnia, irritability, and more. Sophie was unconcerned.

And she and Stan weren't hitting it off. Their views of life, their humor, his wealth and standing in the legal community—her beauty and sweetness should have melded their souls.

Stan complained that the pain medications didn't touch his discomfort even after I increased the dose of Demerol to 150 mg IM every four hours. Stan was a fussy kind of guy, and I didn't give his complaints much credence. Yet his carping caught my attention when he told me the nighttime injections worked fine. Those shots produced a deep mental haze and adequate analgesia. The discrepancy between the effectiveness of the morning and evening medications took me a while before I understood.

# TEN

People with vasculitis were sick, and Sophie was just in a mood. All the annoying little things became big-time issues—her shoes that *clicked-clacked*, my gum chewing, her public displays of affection bringing unwanted attention from the studs at the bars, her stares back at them, the near-fisticuffs, her expensive red wine choices, my rosé selections, the singsong voice she used when ordering dinner; Sophie and I chipped at each other about perceived and real faults instead of having fun.

The university pathologist was pleased to review the skin biopsy with me. The microscope contained six separate heads spaced around a solid wood rectangle table. It was a teaching instrument that offered simultaneous participation by the students and young doctors with the professors.

"The inflammation is sparse and nondescript, with a few white cells here and there," Dr. Wong, the pathologist, lectured me, demonstrating the findings with the microscopes built-in white pointer. "A small-vessel vasculitis is the likeliest possibility, but the inflammation is deeper and more discrete than usual," he said, slipping his steel-rimmed glasses back on.

"Dr. Wong, what did the polarizing view disclose?" I asked, catching the doctor by surprise. Sophie didn't have vasculitis. So uncommon, and so unlikely to only manifest as symmetrical skin lesions on the legs. Dr. Wong smiled at me. "Good question, let's look," he said without rancor and inserted the polarizing plates into the microscope. Similar to our polarized sunglasses, these lenses allow light, which is ordinarily multidirectional, to exit in only one direction. When two polarizing plates were perpendicular to one another, light will not enter the eye and the background remained dark.

Strings of bright specks embedded in Sophie's tissue specimen shone through the otherwise black background of the microscope. Crystalline foreign material present deep in the skin biopsy would allow the light to escape the polarizing plate restrictions. Sophie's skin lesions were explained. Her symmetrically placed lesions on the anterior thighs were within reach of self-inoculation. Her erratic behavior, so unlike my extroverted beauty, and Stan's inability to find pain relief when Sophie was attending him—Sophie was injecting herself with hospital narcotics and substituting saline or something else for Stan and other patients. They were suffering and she was suffering.

My dear Sophie, more generous than Eppie to Silas Marner, lovelier than Elizabeth Taylor in *Raintree County*, more patient than Fiona from Brigadoon, was ill and vulnerable. Was it our messing around with others? Had I forgotten to say that I cared? When did I last bring her flowers?

We met after her shift for a quick coffee in the cafeteria. I told Sophie about the new pathology findings. Dr. Wong was sending an amended pathology report to her doctor describing foreign material present in the biopsy with the new diagnosis of factitial inflammation. Head down and angry, she understood the implications. "You bastard," she yelled, her voice fading away with hoarseness. "What right did you have looking at my biopsy and coming up with that shit?"

"I love you, Sophie. I'll tell the chief that I took the medicine and sold it to make ends meet, but you need help. Let me get it for you. The lesions will heal if you stop abusing yourself, and Dr. Gershon would be willing to see you. I can talk to her, you're hurting yourself and you can't help it."

"Fuck you, Ted, I'll take care of myself. I'll be okay. I'm seeing the nursing chief first. They already know there's a problem. The pharmacy supervisor reported a shortage of Demerol, and I have an appointment with the head of nursing."

"Sophie, I'm sorry. It's my fault isn't it? I love you."

Crying! I had only seen it once before and that during Gary Cooper's ultimate sacrifice for Ingrid Bergman and her comrades in *For Whom the Bell Tolls,* and that was Sophie with a brief sob, more a catch in the throat, one or two tears, a hiccup, nothing more. Cooper only a few minutes left to live, only hours after lovemaking that had moved the earth, and Sophie cried.

"Would it help any, if we got engaged?" I blurted. "You know how much you mean to me."

"Jesus, Ted, that's not how it's done, but thanks," and she stopped, brushed away her tears, and laughed. "Hold me, some more." And I did, and her wet cheek merged with mine and we held each other tighter, rocking together, more meaningful than a two-step dance to "Unchained Melody," the Al Hibbler version, our names whispered to one another. I followed her out of the cafeteria entranceway until she told me she was fine.

Mrs. B walked over and placed her arms around me. "Even big-shot doctors get jilted sometimes. You'll find someone else, maybe not as pretty as Nurse Sophie for sure. Perhaps if you were a little quieter, wore a tie without spaghetti stains, and attended the Emily Post classes I mentioned to you, this wouldn't have happened."

"Thanks Mrs. B," I told her and left it at that. Sophie's problem was private, and what Emily Post classes was Mrs. B talking about?

Relieved of her responsibilities and suspended, Sophie was not fired, and that was fine, since good nurses were in short supply. Hopefully, her addiction would be amenable to treatment. Sophie's competent care-giving was widely recognized and appreciated. Once she was enrolled in a drug rehabilitation program, she would be treated with methadone and required to see Dr. Gershon, my psychiatrist. Life was a continuum and sometimes even circular.

Why did Sophie develop a drug dependence? Craving for narcotics was nearly impossible to stop and Sophie had access to all of them. Our conversations were open and probing, but loaded with speculation and ignorance.

After the consultation with Dr. Gershon and the nursing chief, Sophie decided that a change of venue made sense and she flew to Florida to continue treatment and stay with relatives. A good decision, she was making progress with therapy, but she needed time for herself, and in Florida her problems would not be shared with everyone at our hospital.

❖ ❖ ❖

I joined Sophie. Chicago Midway to Washington D.C. to Fort Lauderdale, all easy flights, room to stretch my legs and sleep—the sleep of the just or was it the damned? Ignored by the stewardesses and my fellow passengers, I was spared mystery food and salesmen providing counsel about the value of term insurance.

The overhead announcement made right before takeoff that my seat cushion could be used as a flotation device in case of a water landing was the only worry. The machinations of extracting the seat cushion, the very same one that I was sitting on, coupled with a mad rush toward the exit door as we crashed into the ocean just east of the airport scrambled my peace.

The car rental people proved obstinate. After a long wait for service, they informed me that they had run out of rental cars, in spite of my confirmed reservation for a compact sedan, either a Pontiac Tempest or a Mercury Comet. Not enough of them had been returned, and it would be a wait and since I wasn't a club member or frequent rental user or something, most of the stiffs standing behind me in line would be awarded cars long before me. Although outwardly polite, quite truthfully, none of the transactions the agents handled were handled with fairness or dignity.

I joined the bums on the bench outside and sat around with the afternoon sun spreading joy on my face, my legs outstretched, savoring the warmth. Florida girls stepped over me, in shorts, or halters, or thin white cotton dresses, waiting for lovers or husbands, their happiness energizing my Midwestern spirits. Waiting around this airport wasn't so bad, and I was proud of my patience. Dr. Gershon would be told how adeptly I handled the frustration.

Sophie lived with her aunt, nowhere near the beach, but sun, warmth, and humidity spread itself generously on this part of Florida. My motel, Triple A, its name, and not likely its rating, was a gift from Harry and my mother, who sent me cash gifts, allowing me to afford these whims, for no reason, just because I was their son. I didn't tell them I soon might have major legal expenses for a murder defense. Their delight in their doctor child didn't need tarnishing during this, the most important year of my training.

Sophie worked odd hours at the local county hospital, on probation status, and administering narcotics only under supervision. She was already a star attraction for the young medics, and the middle-aged and older ones, too, for that matter—being tall, blonde, naturally slinky, and endowed with soft lips, provided a running start in attracting friends. And Sophie was transforming back into her smiley self. Only momentary afternoon spells exposed the remnants of her shakiness. There were never easy answers to the quirks and vagaries that shadowed dependence, and physical closeness and quiet were the only remedies I was allowed to offer.

The dampness and warmth steaming up from newly laid sidewalks mixed with the tropical decay invigorated our senses, relaxed us, and lowered our guard. The late-morning sun bursting through the low-passing clouds spread delight, and we would swim or nap or both. Whiling away the hours in this beautiful world proved more pleasant than confronting my life's craziness. But the latter couldn't be ignored forever.

"Sophie dearest, I need to speak to you about something important," I said, sorry to puncture the serenity. We sat on the cushioned lounge chairs by the motel's pool, the daily newspaper and pulp fiction tucked under us, folded between the mattress and the metal frame, our hands sticky with the suntan lotion we wordlessly spread over each other. Two children, brother and sister, monitored by grandmother, splashed around the shallow end, tossing a rubber ball, periodically crashing on us, their hand-eye coordination lost in giggling and dunking, but not upsetting us. The Atlantic Ocean behind us, the roar of the waves billowed in like clockwork from distant paradises, rhythmic and relaxing, while the sun enveloped us. It was the right moment.

"You know about Tim's Schmidt's death, Betty's husband?" I asked, waiting for Sophie's attention, repeating my question, only louder now until she looked up from her reverie, flashing a fake smile directed somewhere near me, and nodded yes.

"I shot him," I said. "He was a bad guy, a murderer, a thug. He sent the two goons after me to break my knee and puncture my lung." I reached for Sophie's hand, waving goodbye with my other to grandmother who was gathering her charges for a snack back at the motel's diner. "And the shitty thing is that no one seemed to care about what happened to Betty. She counted on me. She should have responded to my treatment, she should be home reading to her children right now, or sitting by a pool watching them play like grandmother over there. Betty was ill, but not fatally ill." Sophie understood the distinction.

"No one seemed to care but me," I repeated, my throat tightening, making me hoarse. "So I shot him."

Sophie was half-listening. Usually, I was the quiet one. Sophie panicked at the least pause in human conversation, but now said not a word.

"I'm listening, Ted." She finally spoke, the Florida morning shadows sweetening her expression. "And I don't believe you. You may want to slug it out with the bad guys, but you don't kill people. And if you did, I don't want to know about it. Jesus, Ted, I'm in a ten-step or whatever program for my problems, and I just can't deal with much more." And with that, she leaned over and muffled my mouth with her palm, playing a catchy tune with her fingers for a few seconds, her effort to halt conversation before returning to Mickey Spillane.

"I was a criminal once," she said. "It was in our fourth-grade drama production. I ran into the on-stage bakery shop dressed as a robber in a mask with a plastic gun, and shouted, 'This is a holdup. Give me a chocolate layer cake and step on it!' and the bakery attendant, my drama-class classmate and best friend, placed the cake on the floor and stepped on it. So I shot her. Sorry Ted, I think I've told you that story before."

Maybe she was right. How much good can come from sharing a felony? The guilt, satisfaction, dismay, appointment in Hades, all mixed together, were mine; they belonged to me and might better stay only between me and God.

We raced across the length of the pool, our daily challenge, and even allowing her a head start, I still won, collecting the chlorine-suffused winner's kiss that banished confessional thoughts.

Sophie's aunt had obtained her real estate license and showed us the future. Palm trees being dragged here and planted there. Hotels and restaurants catering to the sun-starved northerners and Europeans were being constructed along the beach, catching the sunrise and the all-day breezes. The intra-coastal-waterway linked the inland to the sea, providing entrepreneurs with even more opportunities for development.

We danced the last night. Sophie didn't need a partner; she swayed to her own rhythm, brimming with grace and restless energy. "Sure, dancing is important," Sophie told me, one hand in mine, the other stroking my cheek, vestiges of my old Sophie. "But if you really want to please me, actually please girls in general, get us something to wear to parties. Something that lasts, something important—okay, the absolute bottom line is, girls want shoes."

We slurped the tropical drinks, listening to the music and her wisdom, my hands restlessly playing with the toothpick umbrellas impaling the maraschino cherries and orange slices, sword-fighting with them, right hand versus left, good versus evil, the outcome always in doubt, as I pondered my deeds, hoping my subconscious would choose correctly.

The music was slow and sweet, the saxophonist with a smooth voice interspersed with mellow playing. He was the reed instrumentalist Chet Baker. The lead singer, smiling and pointing at the regulars, acknowledged their praise, while caressing the old-fashioned upright microphone and stand she dragged around with her, her own dance lover, as she purred velvet melodies to her crowd.

I kissed Sophie's hand, tasting her fortune lines in her delicious palm, while we danced back to the motel room. Kisses and laughter in the street, in the hallway, and in the elevator, we paused only for hugs, and joyful greetings to the soda machine noisily vibrating outside my door.

The Florida dampness filled every corner of my room; the overhead fan layered the thick air over our skin. The queen-sized bed was high off the floor, clean and empty except for a taut white cotton sheet faded from too many industrial washings, and two pillows neatly stacked at the head—my ear pressed deep into Sophie's left breast, listening to her heart pumping and relaxing, unsure whether I was hearing her happiness or mine.

I hugged Sophie gently where the wounds had been and kissed the barely visible scars, fading away too quickly, unlikely to provide a permanent memory of her misdeeds. Our alcohol-suffused lovemaking playing out in slow motion magnified the pleasure of touches and tastes. There wasn't a part of her that wasn't familiar. Shakespeare was mistaken. He got it wrong. Sophie, not Juliet, was the sun.

I left for home the next morning, as the rising sun curled its gnarled fingers through the wooden slats covering the Triple A motel windows. It had been a storybook kind of week with Sophie slowly becoming her old self, the sunshine and warmth too inviting for her to return home. I promised to write and telephone every chance I had. But we were never again the same.

# ELEVEN

## *Life Goes On*

I took the tunnel. The precipitation shuffled between a drizzle and a downpour and rain always turned my hair fluffy. The tunnel to Psychiatry was new and solid. When the Russkies nuke the Gary-Chicago industrial complex, I'll hunker down there. More importantly, the graffiti lining the white walls was borderline grammatical and occasionally pleasing.

I don't mind trekking to Psychiatry, the hospital was big and everywhere you go you were still around, but Psychiatry was close, and orderly, like the military, the chain of command precise, and the medical resident king. Although today, I thought of myself more as Merlin, summoning up graciousness for the Sunday afternoon pre-electroshock-therapy clearance.

Convulsive therapy was the treatment of choice for too many conditions: rowdy, noncompliant, anorexic, and tearful. *Bam*, the brain exploded into chaos, primary colors, drum and bugle corps, flag waving and fireworks, all in anticipation of the sadness or bizarreness disappearing in slow, hopeful steps. But a lot of other things disappear, too. Gone are the memories of flaxen-haired girls and kisses on late spring days.

Sometimes with electroshock therapy you forget your entire adolescence, never mind flaxen-haired girls.

They knew me here. The potassium a little low, or the electrocardiogram with flattened T waves and I canceled the entire shebang. Even the crazies have gentle memories. I wouldn't have ordered the thing in the first place, but then Psychiatry wasn't a democracy.

The chief of psychiatry would corner me and I would nod my head like an automaton, as if believing his verisimilitudes. "Ted," he'd say, "our imperfect universe seeks equilibrium and not necessarily cures. Psychiatry remains a Newtonian world. Relativity will come later."

"Mr. Winterfeld, Harold?" I asked. No last names in this place. The door unlocked and Harold paced the floor, which was a lot better in my estimation than lying face down in bed and sobbing.

"I'm Dr. Ted, and I'm here to clear you for the procedure tomorrow." The room needing painting, the sole window was fused closed, shatter-proof glass distorting the daylight into specks of the rainbow, light from overhead fluorescents emitting that annoying buzz, just loud enough to further drive you batty.

"*Procedure*" is the euphemism for electrodes being belted around the skull, a three-pronged plug placed into an AC outlet, the cord winding its way into a battery housed in a bland and not unfriendly appearing brass-colored metal box rolled in and out of rooms on four wooden coasters, and an on-off switch with a dial for magnitude, low to high. The apparatus absent only Disney characters, Goofy perhaps. It's Underwriters Laboratory approved; I always search for the UL label.

An attached tray protrudes from the console stocked with jelly that conducts electrons and sticks to the scalp, an invention rivaling airline reclining seats, a plastic mouthpiece, please no fractured teeth, and emergency instructions, for I guess emergencies. Press "on," and *zap*, there it was, an excellent, four-star tonic-clonic seizure, and *voilá*, a docile and contented Harold.

I scanned Harold's wrist ID band. The antithesis of depressed, Harold's pleased for the company, dancing feet, humming from *Aida*, the *Grand March*, now and then stopping to blow the trumpet riffs with a tight fist placed like a horn over his mouth. He's not the typical shock therapy recipient, and yes, it was the correct Harold.

Where was down-in-the-mouth Auntie Maude, children not telephoning, cat run away, tires flat, wine bottles empty, and on and on, the usual ComEd recipient?

"Examine away, Doctor, and what do you think of my tango?" His words accompanied by a little foot-shuffling. "Arthur Murray Dance Studio on Broadway near Lawrence, ask for Dolores, tell her Harold, the sheik of Araby sent you," now gamely singing the tune of the same name that was more likely written for Rudolph Valentino than Harold. "Dolores will be at my all-better, welcome-home party and you're also invited. Guess who else is coming?"

It's best not to enter into their fantasies and hopes. You don't want to reinforce craziness. My job was to be sure Harold survived the electricity. The neurologic examination was normal: reflexes symmetric, sensation intact, optic nerves healthy, no tremors, oriented to time, place, and person. The consent form for the electro-convulsive therapy signed with what appeared to be his handwriting.

"Harold," I told him, "your physical examination and laboratory values are disgustingly normal and I have no reason not to okay the medical clearance for the procedure, unless you have a change of heart. And I'll be honored to attend any *rocking* party you throw."

By Tuesday, Harold would likely have forgotten me and any celebration he'd concocted.

"Eleanor G, she's coming and you won't guess who she is," Harold continued, shifting from one foot to another. "Refreshments, Cole Porter songs, dancing, Eleanor G, and Doctor, I can tell by just looking at you that you need a 'Harold Party.'"

My head bobbing and my hand waving goodbye didn't stop the mania, and I didn't want to be impolite. I remained standing at the door. I have good instincts about people and I liked this guy.

"Eleanor Geisman, of course, the girl next door, my dance partner, you'll have to find your own date," Harold told me. "If Dolores doesn't suit you, maybe phone that cute little—"Yes! We Have No Bananas" girl, from Brazil. You know the one with the fruit hat, platform shoes, and the "Chico-Chico" song and dance."

I knew exactly who Harold meant, having had a crush on her myself but I wasn't going to be the bearer of bad tidings. I hate bad news. Carmen Miranda never sang "Yes! We Have No Bananas," and worse still, she had slipped into the great beyond a few years ago.

Tuesday, I walked over to see Harold. I skipped viewing the actual procedure. Observing one of them earlier in my career had provided enough disturbances in spite of the blankets and straitjacket and pillows thoughtfully provided to prevent broken bones.

Harold was walking the halls, not appreciably worse for the wear, as best as I could see. "I'm here to check up on you," I told him. No aide or nurse shadowed him.

"He's taking his medicine real good now," Tiny, the weightlifting orderly, assured me.

"Never better," Harold said. "And, Doctor, let me save you time," he added. "Today's Tuesday, 7 from 100 is 93, 7 from 93 is 86, etc., etc., the president is Kennedy, our senators are Douglas and Dirksen. How am I doing? Want more?" he boasted.

He was smart and quick, Mensa material, and I was pleased, very pleased, and I told him that, and we hugged. Confident, feet still, and he was quiet in between the showing off.

I showed him the picture I had cut out from the *Daily News*, the movie section, a showing of *Little Women* starring Eleanor Geisman, aka June Allyson, in the role of Jo, the spirited one, the sister who finds romance.

Of course, I'd had to perform a little research about Eleanor G.

"Your favorite," I told him, "for the coming home party"—my index finger circled her face, "Eleanor Geisman," I said.

"Who's that" he asked.

# PART FIVE

# ONE

## *Late Spring 1962*

Sergeant Esposito and I met for dinner. His request, no reason tendered, but I read the command in his tone when he telephoned. The neighborhood just east of the medical school was an enclave of old Italy. The well-kept-up older homes and gardens showcased vegetable plots with too many varieties of summer squash and tomatoes. Dotted on the inside commercial street were family restaurants offering an assortment of delicacies as long as they were Italian. The pasta with red sauce was the main attraction for the students, but Puglian, Venetian, and even Italian-Austrian delicacies were offered for connoisseurs such as the sergeant and me, plus, the glorious red wines for sipping that matched our appetites.

We settled into the back booth of a quiet family restaurant adorned with the whitest of tablecloths and thick cloth napkins spotted correctly on the left side of the dinner plate lying underneath the panoply of different-sized and tined-forks. No wax-coated-chianti bottles desecrated the walls with candles protruding from their mouths like stale cigars seeking a Zippo lighter. I found myself sitting up straight, hands in my lap, head up, accommodating to the refinement. The waitress, an Italian Unification War widow, recommended the spaghetti carbonara, the evening's special. "No cream," she said. "Americans use cream," she repeated, staring at me. "And pancetta not bacon," distorting her face at the idea of somebody not using the air-dried pork belly cured in salt and spices, and with that she kissed George on the cheek and flashed a skeptical wave at me. "After spaghetti, I bring veal."

Anthony, the owner's son delivered the martinis himself, dry and cold, and then the house red poured into juice glasses. I felt at home.

After multiple *salutis* and glass-clicking, and following the spaghetti and lightly breaded veal smothered in spicy marinara sauce, mixed with scallions, sautéed onions, sun-dried tomatoes, red peppers and more than a trace of amaretto, but before the dessert of cream-filled cannoli, George cleared his throat and asked me without fanfare—"Do you know a Bill Tomczak?"

Maybe I shouldn't have felt so comfortable.

"This guy Tomczak purchased a pistol similar to the one used by the mob hit that knocked off Tim Schmidt. And what's so weird about it, is that our gun owner Tomczak is, *kaput, morto, martwy*, dead. Now how does a dead guy buy a gun? Crazy, huh?" George shoveled the food down, with only a brief glance toward me.

"Hey, George, this cannoli is good, and where do they find coffee this rich? I need to tell Mrs. B about it."

"Dead for *months*," the sergeant continued, an unleashed player piano programmed for persistent annoyance.

"I met his widow, nice-looking lady, by the way, and surprise, surprise, she knows and speaks highly of her dear friend Dr. Ted."

Then a pause to enjoy the coffee and dessert, mouth still working, silent, but only for a moment.

"I think you know all the good-looking women in the city," George continued. "Have you ever considered setting up a dating service for old cops like me?"

No comment from me. I remained a passenger in this conversation.

"Mrs. Tomczak tells me that Bill, her husband, her *deceased* husband, Mr. Tomczak, never owned any guns, disliked them a lot, actually.

"You're right about the coffee, Doc, it's Colombian, not blended with anything else, and roasted slow. Be patient when brewing it, that's the key—heat it slowly. Keep the pot covered tight so the flavor stays in. I'll have some packed for you."

"George, you're amazing. You have time to be a gourmet, a coffee aficionado, an excellent judge of women, an enemy of bad people, and an all-around good guy, and you share it with me. I know Mrs. B is crazy about you, and if you want I can mention your culinary desires to her, or to Amy Tomczak."

My little soliloquy meant nothing; nothing stops a policeman when he's on a roll.

"It's funny about coincidences, Doc."

*Jesus, George, get off this subject*, I complained to myself.

"A guy dies at your hospital, well you work at a big place, yet you know his wife, so you must have known Bill, Mr. Tomczak, the guy with the gorgeous wife. Did I say that already? That's right, you even know her first name. That's amazing by itself. Amy is it? And this guy, dead as a doornail, buys the exact same kind of gun used to kill your nemesis. Life is filled with riddles; just like right now, a clean-cut, excellent doctor, trying his best to do good in this world, saving lives one at a time and enjoying wonderful food and wine with some run-of-the mill cop attempting to earn his meager salary. And here we are, both sharing our admiration of beauty and the need to keep our streets safe."

The restaurant was getting noisier as the downtown suits accompanied by their secretaries began to arrive, their presence announced with winks and laughter. The importance of levity when performing evening stenography had previously escaped me. And no need to scan the restaurant populace before entering. Wives or children were unlikely to dine here alone on a weeknight.

"The higher-ups crossed you off as a suspect," George continued, over the background hum. "The pristine gun we found in your apartment was a brilliant piece of work. And you would think that we had better things to do than trying to find out who killed the slime ball Tim. But what can I tell you? The case is open again. So if you get any ideas, call me."

I saluted my good friend George and thanked the owner for the wonderful food.

I'd call Stan Glicke and obtain advice about my life and my new, but difficult-to-figure out adversary, the sergeant.

Maybe it was time to talk to Howard.

# TWO

Actually, Howard brought it up himself.

We were on call. The storage room connecting the rear of the cafeteria with the auditorium housed an upright piano that could be rolled into either place. That had never happened as best as I could remember. The spindly wooden wheels were encased by spider webs spun during the Harding administration. Musty and damp there, the acoustics stank, the walls tiled with walnut-colored plastic and spotted with age, reminiscent of the knotty-pine playrooms that children were banished to after late-summer dinners, stacked with yellowed boxes of Monopoly sets, checkers, and incomplete 1000-piece puzzles. No *Park Place* or *Boardwalk* this place, and not comforting like the cafeteria, but there were chairs, the piano, and quiet.

There was a peculiar trance at that time of day. Procedures had been completed, the ER was caught up, and if Ponce de Leon had settled permanently in America, we'd be taking siestas now like the rest of the civilized world instead of gabbing and singing.

*Now in the Chapel where Laura prays*
*For her poor Tommy, who passed away*
*It was just for Laura he lived and died*
*Alone in the chapel she can hear him cry*

"What's going on big fellow?" Howard asked. He can't leave a piano alone. He was singing and playing. It was why we were here, rather than fighting with Mrs. B in the cafeteria.

I was slouched down, my head resting against the splat of the wooden chair, not singing along, and Howard knew something was up. Few of us tell everything we know to others, even our loved ones. My Tim Schmidt secret, would I be exposing a weakness? Would the recounting of my deed only satisfy a narcissistic need?

"You're ready to burst out with something and it's been that way for weeks," Howard paused for a moment, eyes closed in concentration, communing with his own musical world.

"Is it about Sophie? God I miss her. Give her a call, will you. And Estelle, for chrissakes, she's engaged; she's not on the market, so to speak, and have you heard the latest news about Fineglass?"

"Fineglass? No, nothing about Dr. Danger has crossed my path, and Sophie, dear Sophie, and for that matter Estelle—I miss them," I whined.

"Guess what I played for my first recital?" Howard asked, music directing his thoughts. "I was seven, the youngest in the music class, and the other captives were tinkling Haydn and Mozart. My parents were there, so proud of me. I bowed low during my introduction, then three pieces, one right after another. My dad loved classical music, our Philco always tuned to Beethoven or Handel. It was 'Macaroni Cha Cha' followed by 'Please No Bees' and then 'Pumpkin Boogie' by Faber, not C.P.E. Bach, my contribution to the entertainment. No hug, I received a slap on the top of my head, and double the practice time and you see how well it worked because twenty years later and thousands of dollars thrown to a gaggle of music instructors and here I am playing this classic.

*Tell Laura I love her*
*Tell Laura I need her*

It was funny how well Howard could sing, and play the piano, be a doctor, and worry about me. He was the king of the world.

*Tell Laura not to cry*
*My love for her will never die*

We sang together in harmony, thriving on musical tragedy.

*Tell Laura not to cry*
*My love for her will never die*

"I'm in the ER, and we paged Surgery for a GI bleeder," Howard told me. "Fineglass answers, but he can't come down right away, he's polishing his white bucks and then they have to dry, he tells the head nurse. She's as pissed as the rest of us, as we infuse an extra pint of blood into the patient and hatch this once-in-a-lifetime prank. Of course Fineglass doesn't get it.

'Dr. Fineglass,' she says. 'You've heard of the Fulbright Scholarship for academic merit and leadership skills, you know, the one named after the senator from Arkansas?

"Meanwhile, Fineglass is nodding his head like Howdy Doody on coke and playing with his semicircle specs on the glass chain hanging from his neck. Maybe he's heard of the J. William Fulbright Scholarship, maybe not, he's busy searching his reflection in a mirror, trying out a smile, straightening his bow tie and strands of hair, his shoes glowing brighter than those atomic tests run in New Mexico.

"'Well,' she says, 'we have our very own special award for you. It comes from our collective hearts,' and Nurse-in-Charge Janetta hands him an official-looking document.

"'Thanks,' he says, momentarily perking up. 'The Half-Bright Award,' he reads it aloud and says: 'Neat, let me phone Mom to tell her about it, thanks, and here sometimes I thought you guys weren't always on my side.'"

The mood wasn't exactly what I had hoped for, what with the Fineglass story and Laura and Tommy and their troubles, but my murder of Tim would go down easier if I could share it with Howard. I had thought about it. I had to get it off of my mind. I was ready to burst out with confession and Howard would understand. It was too late to help Laura and her problems with clumsy Tommy, who had crashed his racecar.

*No one knows what happened that day how his car overturned in flames*

"This has to remain between us, the stuff I'm telling you," I said to Howard. "You could be an accessory to a crime." My concerns were not as pitiful as Laura's and much less than that of Tommy's.

"Ted, if you want to borrow the cheerleading skirts and pom-poms for your next date with Sophie and you want to ask Jane for hers, go for it. It'll be more fun than Sophie wearing a Girl Scout uniform or a Brownie outfit—alright, never mind, if it's the latter, I don't even want to hear about it. One other thing, tell me about your church, was it like my temple, some of the time spent thinking about God and standing and sitting and reciting, but mostly spent dreaming about beating up the bully sitting in the third row or accidently brushing against the breasts of the young mother sitting next to you?"

I was not smiling.

"I killed Tim Schmidt, and only Sergeant Esposito knows it, and now you do too. I had two guns. The police found the one I set up for them and that one had never been fired," I told Howard.

I could have been forecasting the long term weather for Death Valley as far as Howard was concerned.

"George Esposito, the cop I turned to for assistance, realizes that I'm the perp, but I don't know if he can prove it or if he even cares. Believe me," I added, "it's unsettling."

"Hey, man I knew it all along, the murder I mean. It's not new. I read your soul. Tim deserved it. You did the right thing. It took guts. I couldn't have done it. But you and I, damn it, we remember every death. We can't help it. Then when a patient dies who shouldn't have, too young, not that ill, it makes us stay awake at night, our brain working overtime while we twist in bed for hours. Betty murdered and so young, you'll never be able to let that go. You had to do something."

Howard turned to the piano for just a moment, concentrating on several chords, joining Laura and Tommy.

"Even your gun purchase took machismo," he said, turning to look at me. "Jane and I and the entire wedding party will wear prison stripes if need be. You're still my best man. They're the same as wives anyway, best men, right? You can't testify against them in court, like a husband-and-wife confidentiality thing, so you can tell me everything. That's legal stuff and I'm sure it's written down somewhere."

My smile was thin.

"Big guy," Howard continued, "I'm on your side. Move on to better things. Let Stan Glicke handle your defense. Jesus, he owes you favors, and if you need cash, count on me and Jane."

A bear hug, and I was near tears after unloading my atavistic impulses. I felt better already, clumsy with relief. Howard sat back down on the piano bench, me nearly falling onto him. I wouldn't unload on anyone else. Maybe killing Tim Schmidt had been ordained and beyond the bailiwick of mortals. The isolation of the storage room, the privacy, no access to the elements, no snow or wind, the quiet confession, Howard offering advice, it was all a balm for my conscience. Thanks for listening, buddy.

*But as they pulled him from the twisted wreck*
*With his dying breath they heard him say*
*Tell Laura I love her*

The on-call-pagers were complaining, the annoying vibration that brings no joy, the living not the dead were beckoning and they demanded answers.

# THREE

One patient after another, the Cardiology month was a marathon, our day never ending until well past sundown. There were too many fathers and uncles having heart attacks too early in their lives leaving widows in austere circumstances. Meat in portions large enough to satisfy big cat carnivores, little exercise, constant stress, undiagnosed diabetes mellitus, and inadequately treated hypertension took its toll in spite of our well-meaning ministrations.

Howard was part of this rotation, two smug senior residents at the top of their learning curve, happy and hyper in spite of the exhausting schedule. Incessantly talking medicine, quizzing each other on mundane facts, our heads thrown back, fists up in the air, shouting "yes," with our correct responses.

Certification in the specialty of Internal Medicine required a written examination scheduled during the third month of our future training at the university, Howard in his GI fellowship and me in the hematology laboratory. The test entailed two full days of concentrated nitpicking over indistinct X-ray pictures, blurred photographs of skin lesions and blood smears, interspersed with case reports describing medical events occurring once every cicada outburst. We loved it. Obscure questions were our forte, and correct responses were as rewarding as outguessing the chief.

For unaccountable reasons, several bright residents would fail the examination, and that kept us compulsively studying. The unpleasantness of retaking the examination included the humiliation of being known as a flunkey. Only the chief and the unlucky resident received the failure notice, but rumor spread fast in our backstabbing community. At the following year's examination locale, where you unobtrusively showed up for the second attempt to pass, *in mufti,* of course, your junior colleagues with their well-honed instincts, taking the examination for the first time, boisterously surrounded you in spite of you slouching low in the last row on the left, the side with the burnt-out ceiling light, and wearing your shades, dark clothes, and a baseball cap, rim down to your nose. False greetings were rendered, your name shouted to the world and everybody became cognizant of your failure.

Howard and I were too smart for that to happen to us. We were the kings of our team, sharper even than the cardiology fellows and of course the younger residents and students. "What are seven causes of renal failure in multiple myeloma?" we shouted. Questions of that ilk we could answer in a flash, and we willy-nilly tossed out these nuggets of wisdom to our associates.

Then it happened. One of the cardiology fellows, who thought he could compete with us, presented a patient we were seeing in consultation. All of us standing around the bedside, the curtains pulled around the poor soul, our desultory attempt at privacy while we talked about Mr. Sanders as if he was traveling to a better place.

Wide-open aortic insufficiency in this previously healthy fifty-year-old man was discovered serendipitously during an examination for fever and neck pain. There was no silence in between the heart's *lub* and *dub*—the quiet replaced by noise, a rumble, loud at first, and then softening. Mr. Sanders's aortic valve didn't close properly and a sizeable portion of the rich oxygenated blood meant for distribution throughout the body flowed back into the left side of the heart and set the aortic valve in vibration.

"Doctors," Mr. Sanders began, glancing around at all of us, frustration modulating his voice, "you're always listening to my heart, but my biggest problem is sleep. I can't sleep. Can't anyone tell me why?"

The cardiology fellow didn't give a shit about this guy's sleep. He only listened to hearts, but Howard and I cared. What did sleep have to do with Mr. Sanders's heart unless he became orthopneic, short of breath when lying down? And that wasn't the case.

"I can't sleep because my ears hurt when they touch the pillow." Mr. Sanders offered the pearl. "I can't lie on my side because these hurt," he said, pulling his pinnae, the outer part of the ear, and wincing at the same time.

Howard and I nudged each other, doors had opened, cardiology became fun, and the Nobel Prize in Medicine might well be within our reach. Mr. Sanders's ears were red, tender and swollen, now that we actually looked at them.

"These other areas also hurt, don't they?" I asked the unfortunate Mr. Sanders, gently squeezing his nose just below the nasal bone and at the front of his neck over the trachea, apologizing about the discomfort.

Suggesting to the team that we talk outside, I thanked Mr. Sanders, who was still lying in wonderment, worried about what was in store for him. "It's a wondrous thing that so many talented doctors are interested in your well-being," I said, while we opened the curtains and exited.

"Great patient, Doctor," we informed the cardiology fellow. "Thanks for sharing him with us plebeians."

"Relapsing polychondritis is such an uncommon disease," Howard said.

"And so often missed, even by excellent clinicians," I added.

"It's an autoimmune disease," Howard said, "with antibodies directed against cartilage. That's why all the places that Dr. Ted touched, the nose, the trachea, and the ears were tender. They all contain cartilage."

"Mr. Sanders may also have arthritis because the joints become inflamed, what with all the cartilage there, too," I added with a straight face. "Anti-inflammatory medication should be started soon. It might diminish the aortic valve insufficiency. As all of you know, those valves are rich in cartilage and are prime targets for the antibodies. Mr. Sanders telling us about his sleep problems and the pain when his ears touched his pillow clinched the diagnosis.

"Great patient! We're ready to move on, unless there are any questions?" Howard and I stared at the cardiologist after our explanations, our act honed to perfection. After all, we'd been performing together for four years of medical school and almost three years of the IntMed program.

Relapsing polychondritis, Mr. Sanders's illness, was poorly understood and difficult to treat. Antibodies were directed toward cartilage, the pliable white stuff, the gristle that lies between bones, the material that shapes our noses, our windpipes, and the outer part of our ears. Mr. Sanders had consulted several doctors, complaining about the ear pain and the swelling, but the condition had been mistaken for cellulitis, a common skin infection.

Howard and I were experts on relapsing polychondritis, which we shortened to "RP" for the edification of our coworkers, since we had read about it several days before. Serendipity for sure, but someone, somewhere, said luck comes to the well-prepared. We imbibed several cold ones that evening celebrating this astonishing stroke of good fortune. At morning report, we spoke in tandem about RP—fact after fact after fact, memorized from our recent reading, but we recited to our colleagues as if that information had resided in our memory bank since birth.

"The diagnosis of RP should be apparent to even the dullest among you," we exclaimed. And I was enthralled about the circumstances allowing our precisely regulated immune system to go awry and attack ubiquitous tissues such as cartilage—more things to discuss with Drs. Brennan and Rhoban.

I didn't forget Mr. Sanders, who unfortunately was a candidate for heart valve replacement, but anti-inflammatory medications prompted pain relief of the ear pain and allowed him to experience deeper sleep.

❖ ❖ ❖

The year was ending. I seemed to be in the good graces of Mrs. Gail and the chief, and except for Sophie remaining in Florida, I was on a roll. Phil was visiting her and thinking about real estate investing with Sophie's aunt. Once the oceanfront property was gone, it was gone, I was told.

"Sophie, date the neurosurgeons or radiologists until we get back together," I told her, but she just laughed. No mention was made about the fate of Tim Schmidt and our motel pool conversation.

I had a full plate—the end-of-the year-hospital-graduation party, reviewing vast amounts of literature for internal medicine boards, organizing my research ideas for a running start at the university, understanding platelet antibodies, and, of course, there was Estelle's wedding.

Dwelling deep in my dreams and erupting at odd and too-frequent occasions were indelible memories of her long legs around my face, her 2:15 a.m.

smell and taste happening to me so fast, like the downward spin of the final grains of sand in an hourglass. "Estelle," I said her name out loud to myself. I wanted to hear its sound.

Joy in reminiscing about my good fortune was tempered by the presence of Sergeant George Esposito waiting for me at morning coffee. Mrs. B buttering the perfectly browned rye-bread toast for him—*gratis*, as she ran to the register to collect the money for my coffee, charging extra for the giant portion although I only had the large cup half-filled because no small containers were to be found.

"Doc, we're dropping the Tomczak/Schmidt thing for now. It just doesn't add up. Do you ever get more information than you can handle? Way too much for tiny-brained cops like me. Sure you do, you must, you're a doctor. Like finding out that the Thanksgiving Day Parade Queen is being treated for a social disease. Her second go-around no less." George paused, but only for a moment. "By the way, the breakfasts here are terrific. I keep on forgetting to tell the guys at the precinct about the good food, the lovely Mrs. B, and the presence of my favorite doctor."

"George, I have to get to work." I was not happy to see my policeman friend, and not mincing words. "Stan Glicke, my lawyer, I believe you know him, he's put some of your buddies in jail although he only has kind words for you, suggests I not talk to policemen. Time to move on, so to speak, so just call me if you have any medical questions I can help you with, especially test results requiring weekly injections of penicillin."

"Dr. Ted,"—he grabbed my arm—"we're friends forever. I'm hurt that you wouldn't want to see me on a regular basis, and yes, I'm here on business, so sit down, be careful, don't spill your coffee on me, and give me your great smile, the one that enchants everyone. Did I tell you that Amy and I had a visit and she talked nonstop about her handsome and smart young doctor? Doc, it's my opinion that she's too old for you, and if you're as brilliant as she claims, why isn't the mister still around?" George was second-guessing my medical expertise.

He told me about the new deal. His last request, if it indeed was a request. It was the quid pro quo for squashing the Tomczak information.

The concatenation of me, Tim Schmidt, and the two thugs, Mr. Big and Mr. Baseball, needed resolution, he said. It involved a package he'd deliver to me, and then some complicated stuff about watching my back and paging him for help at every dark alley crossing.

"Doc, after this is over, we're just friends, cold beers together, barbecue on Sunday afternoons, swimming even. The aboveground pool in my backyard is the centerpiece of the neighborhood." The sergeant spoke with sincerity. "Bond with the good people, the firemen, the city workers, the sewer and garbage guys, men who work hard, folks you can count on when the chips are down. And their wives, you'll love them—stay-at-home, good-looking, smart, God-fearing and good mothers all.

"Hey Doc, I'm not kidding with my speech, we're cut from the same cloth, you and I. We're friends and buddies. Think about the fun we'll share when life settles down." George was sounding very much like my previous adversary, Tim Schmidt, just before his untimely demise. "But I need this one little favor," he said, his voice now laced with a steely timbre.

"George, no packages, no favors, I don't even need to think about it. I'm not part of whatever scheme you're cooking up. I'm a physician, I attend patients, and that's all I do. I can't help you," my hands, flat and low were mimicking the "safe" call by the umpire after the successful steal of second, my words clipped and precise.

Ignoring my baseball re-enactment, the Sergeant continued, his eyes meeting mine, "One of the patrolmen will leave the package at your house. Carry it with you for the next week or so, just in case we screw up. Be alert, although we'll be around to help. Call me anytime; my beeper is always turned on for you. We're a team. Brothers promoting justice in a difficult and crime filled world." This was followed by George's trump card, spoken softly. "*Do this and there will never, ever, be a mention of a doctor with two guns. You have my word.*"

It was there the next day. The phone call from George also, telling me to listen up, that my life depended on it.

I can say something positive about the police. They wrap packages beautifully. All those needy-kids Christmas drives provide expertise with holiday wrapping paper, tight creased corners, and matching ribbon and bows. The special treat was a .38-caliber pistol and I'm an expert on handguns. This one was roughened with use, most likely because of head banging—pistol-whipping, I believe it's called. This pistol had seen adventure. It was loaded with six shells.

The deal involved the two thugs who now seemed part of my life. The rumor on the street had them looking for Tim's murderer, and I was suspect number one. No misdeed was left unpunished in their world. I needed to carry protection. "The mob expects payback," George said over the phone. "No orphan murders riding their books. They know tidy. It's all hearsay, of course, and for the moment all we can do is listen to the streets and keep an eye on you."

"George, how could they tie me to Tim's death? Everyone knows that the gun I had, the one you took from me, was never fired. What's going on? This isn't official police business—the police don't arm civilians." George didn't reply. But I knew the answer. It was staring me in the face and goose bumps were popping up on my extremities quicker than Popeye's forearms after downing a teeming bowl of spinach.

I placed the pistol in my glove compartment along with rubber gloves swiped from the surgery department. No Dr. Ted fingerprints on this weapon. I drove out to the west suburbs for a visit with my pal Big Al and purchased a similar .38-caliber piece. I was not worried that the inscription on my tombstone would read, Two Gun Ted, He Always Packed An Extra." I knew the value of a surfeit of weapons.

I tried this one out on the range in the back of the store, paid in cash, thanked our Founding Fathers for the right to bear arms, and drove home for a good night's sleep, ready to face both the medical and criminal worlds the next day.

And both worlds were quiet. Jane was at a lawyer meeting in St. Louis, Sophie was still in Florida, Estelle, Amy, and Sarah were not with me for a variety of good reasons, the former needing no explanation, the latter three busy with their lives. Howard and I grooved to music, Brubeck and

Desmond, the latter's saxophone rivaling the dry martinis we sipped along with the music: Dave and Paul, Ted and Howard, cool and creative.

# FOUR

Craig Tollen, fifty-two-years old, experienced crushing chest pain, and heart patients arriving in the ER were my responsibility. An ex-professional athlete, he lifted weights and ran hard every morning before sunrise. The pain was blamed on his exercises and multiple eight-minute miles in spite of a worrisome family history. Father, older brother, and uncle were either smitten or dead with coronary artery disease.

Single, after a messy public divorce, Craig needed to maintain a chiseled self if he expected his current soul mate to stick around.

Sitting next to him, she held his hand, long blond hair shifting back and forth, offering expressions of concern. She was able to have found time to paint her lovely face, thicken her eyelashes, add eyeliner, fresh lipstick, and a touch of rouge on cheeks that didn't need touching. "Joy Perfume from Jean Patou, EAU D'hadrien, fifteen-hundred dollars retail," she told me, her accent passable, spreading springtime and libidinous thoughts for the male contingent sharing the emergency room. Fresh, formfitting woolen dress, sweater open in front allowing those confined to this dreary set of rooms and harboring UV light-deprived depression, a chance to partake a bit of sunshine.

Truth be told, I, too would rise at the crack of dawn, tote the weights, and bulk up for the likes of her. "Call me Sandra, Doctor," she was speaking to me, conflating the images of next-door Doris Day and the-other-side-of-the-tracks Lana Turner. Her dark brown eyes did not at all match the color of her shoulder-length hair, as she estimated my future financial worth, testing the waters in case poor Craig didn't make it. It was unlikely that I would receive the stamp of fiduciary fitness, but that didn't diminish my sincere and concerned smile.

Craig had been treated with morphine after his arrival, and the ER doctors had started an intravenous line, taped his ECG and chest X-ray to his cart, and awaited my evaluation for admission to our heart attack unit, while they were off saving lives in people with better outlooks than Craig. The routine blood tests had been sent to the laboratory. Now he was my problem.

The trouble was, Craig's pain hadn't been relieved with the narcotic, and the pain didn't travel down his arm, or up his neck, or settle in the front of his chest, the usual pathways for coronary occlusions. It radiated to his back. There was no response to sublingual nitroglycerin, usually helpful in treating coronary vasospasm. And the ECG was a downer. No ST segment changes, just minimal T wave flattening, too benign for a typical myocardial infarction. I thought about pericarditis, inflammation surrounding the heart, but his heart rate was too slow, and I couldn't hear the scratchy rubbing sound that entity produced.

"Craig, have you had a prior chest X-ray or ECG at our hospital?" I asked, and he mouthed "*X-ray*" and went back to his moaning. I yelled to the ER nurse, "More morphine please, another four milligrams IM stat, and ask the ECG technician to take another tracing. I know, I know, she was just here, tell her sorry about the extra work, but I need it, stat. I want to see if the ECG has changed. And for the moment hold the heart attack unit transfer."

I ran upstairs to Radiology with the new chest X-ray, I had already called Renée, my sweetheart in the filing room, asking her to locate the previous X-rays and bring them to Dr. Burt Brown, the X-ray chief. Renée would be repaid later with coffee and words of endearment. I would tell her how lovely she was, sing to her even, ignoring the crooked teeth, the overbite, and the extra ten pounds ringing her hips.

Dr. Brown was in his office. He didn't like to be bothered by medical residents, and similar to almost everyone else at the hospital, we had a long history. He would yell at us and become angry, reporting us to the chief of medicine for our rowdiness, but before doing that he would read the X-ray and quietly provide his opinion. And it was a thoughtful and expert one. We liked Dr. Brown, and more importantly, we valued his judgment, although the feeling of respect wasn't mutual.

"Dr. Brown, I need your help," I said after knocking once and entering. His secretary did say he was in and alone. "And I'm sorry to barge in," a paean of the more sensitive side of me speaking, but of course I mumbled the sentiment to near-incomprehension.

His stare was derived from Mrs. Gail's repertoire, maybe they were related or attended religious services together, but he held out his hand for the X-ray. Dr. Brown had spent his prime academic life interpreting chest X-rays, and he was willing to forego animosities in order to enlighten me.

I provided Craig's history and told him about the radiation of the pain to the back and the ECG that wasn't classic for a myocardial infarction.

Wordlessly, he examined the X-ray, turned to look at me, but I pre-empted him, pointed to his door, and said, "Renée's bringing the previous examinations. There was one performed here six months ago for cough and fever." That brought a wisp of a smile, and *bang* the door opened right on cue, revealing a smug Renée, helpful as always, carrying the previous X-rays. "Thank you, Renée," I said and blew her a kiss, hoping orthodontia was on this year's schedule.

I owed her many favors throughout the years. She would save the X-ray discards for me, the accidentally obtained double exposures that included the chest and knees on the same film, or the skull X-ray superimposed on an abdomen film, looking very much like a pregnancy, but with a full-sized adult head, no body, resting comfortably in the belly. When our morning report conferences became tedious, as they did so often, I'd place the oddball radiographs on the view board and ask a contemporary to interpret it, receiving interesting and often witty diagnoses.

"There's widening of the mediastinum that's new since the last X-ray. Everything else is unchanged from the previous. Please leave the films here, I'll read them officially," Dr. Brown said, not wanting his less-skilled radiologists to screw up the report with their interpretations.

"Thank you, Dr. Brown. I'm most appreciative of your help, and so will be the patient and his family"—words that usually soothed the good doctor, after which I gently closed his door. Now he couldn't see me use his private phone and dial the page operator.

"Millie, honey, it's Dr. Ted," I said, as if Millie the page operator didn't recognize me after not quite three years of badgering and annoyance. "I want you to page my cardiology attending, the vascular surgeon on call, and the ICU chief, and ask them to either meet me in the ER in five minutes or call me there. It's about a VIP patient. Thanks, dearest."

No comments from Millie, but I could picture her smile directed toward the other operators as she paged the big-shot doctors, humbly delivering the urgent message emanating from a lowly resident whom the bigwigs couldn't ignore, even if they were lecturing at an international conference or sharing coffee time with their inamorata.

Craig was more comfortable now; the extra morphine had provided a token of relief. Sandra was still beautiful. Manny Cohen, my cardiology attending, was at the bedside interpreting the ECG, and the vascular surgeon was inspecting the ceiling, pissed that the chest X-rays were not available, while the ICU chief was on the telephone.

I presented the history of chest pain and the physical examination findings and provided Dr. Brown's interpretation of the X-rays. The two senior physicians were capable of listening to my recitation while keeping Sandra in their line of sight.

Manny listened to the chest and heart, quickly and proficiently. He took charge.

"Craig,"—he was talking to the patient, but his eyes included Sandra—"we all think,"—graciously including me with a sweep of his arm—"that you may have a dissection of the aorta. Of course, we need to perform more testing, but that diagnosis explains the severity of the pain that's radiating to your back, the nonspecific electrocardiogram findings that remain stable, and the current chest X-ray demonstrating a new widening of the aorta. All of those findings would be unusual for a heart attack."

Richard Emit, the vascular surgeon, not wanting to be excluded from the discussion, broke in. "The options are surgery or careful monitoring while we lower your blood pressure in the ICU. This young doctor already has their chief on the phone," he said, acknowledging me with an index finger pointed at my chest. "Your blood pressure is high and I would recommend the latter approach, lowering your blood pressure with medications and being reevaluated in several hours.

"Doctor,"—he pointed at me again, already taking over for Craig, tell the ICU that Craig will be there in one of my beds with Manny being the secondary attending." The lines of authority, normally worked out in private, were being played out right here for our VIP and his guest. Neither of the attending doctors had ever stood so straight and worked their smiles and frowns so beguilingly. Dr. Emit, tall, with blond hair never out of place, an ex-athlete himself, among the royalty of the surgeons, was a commanding presence and proffered trust in everyone he encountered. But it was left for me to tell Craig and Sandra the implications of this life-threatening diagnosis. Manny's office was already offered as a place for Sandra to phone the family and Craig's business associates.

A new intravenous medicine, nitroprusside, efficiently lowered the blood pressure and the ICU chief would have it ready for Craig, who had quietly slipped into sleep from the sedative effects of the morphine.

I organized a team of students to help push Craig to the ICU. The ER nurses phoned in the admission to the admitting office, glad to have Craig and me out of there. It's not a good sign to have white-coated people pushing your gurney, as we cleared the elevator of passengers. "Step aside please, please step aside," spoken with our recently acquired authority that allowed us to arrive at our destination with dispatch.

Craig remained stable with the medical treatment for his dissecting aneurysm. The pain lessened as soon as his blood pressure was lowered. His ECG remained unchanged, and he was scheduled for an X-ray procedure where dye would enter his aorta.

Craig and his family were major donors to the hospital and despite the visiting restrictions in the ICU, he received a stream of well-wishers ranging from the hospital president to my chief of medicine. Everybody was pleased with the prompt diagnosis of the aneurysm made by Manny and the chief of vascular surgery. The X-ray procedure confirmed the diagnosis. What a good hospital we were.

# FIVE

It's justified paranoia that has made me careful about checking the backseat of my automobile, parking in different locations, and searching the rearview mirror at every intersection on my way home. My car was empty, no intruder had taken pity on me and washed and Turtle Wax-ed it; and no one tailed me home sporting a WWII bazooka hanging out their side window aimed at my taillights.

Traffic was light. Our rush hour lasts indefinitely, but tonight traffic flowed. No accidents, no deranged traffic signals, no drawbridges flipped up for the wealthy few with their tall-masted sailing ships heading home to river moorings from the lake and completely stalling traffic, and no sudden torrential cloudbursts that flummoxed cautious drivers. I felt good about Craig. Hopefully, his aneurysm would heal while his blood pressure remained low. Glancing at Sandra had made the workday fly quickly. My personal stock would zenith if she'd be my guest at our year-end party while Craig was recovering.

Sophie wasn't ready to return from Florida, Sarah was traveling to Argentina to visit her beau, Estelle was soon to be married, Amy was backed up with family chores, Mrs. Gail remained married, and Mrs. B had responded to my party invitation by charging extra for the ice cubes I added to my peach-flavored iced tea.

I skillfully maneuvered my too-large Oldsmobile into the narrow parking space, the automobile antiquated for sure, but the power steering worked smoothly. Suffused with the gloss of a successful day, I meandered down the street to my apartment building. Quiet dominated the neighborhood, dinner had been consumed, children were being shepherded to bedrooms wearing their too-snug Dr. Denton's hurriedly snapped closed, and only bedtime stories and good-night prayers remained. The daddy fantasizing about lovemaking, but romance only possible if the stars aligned favorably and the pleading articulated with humility and inventiveness.

That's when I noticed the problem. The light streaming from my corner apartment window was wrong. I leave the three-way bulb on the middle setting, the seventy-five-watt position. I knew exactly how much incandescence it produced. Right now the lamp was too bright, maybe one-hundred or one hundred fifty watts. I forget the wattage of the higher setting.

Everybody knows how unreliable three-way light bulbs are. They burn out regularly. But what happens when that occurs? Do they go dark, or do they shift up to the higher setting? They didn't teach that in medical school. I should have walked over to the drugstore or the telephone booth down the block and called the sergeant, but I'm tough and I have the pistol that George sent me stashed in the glove compartment and under the passenger's seat was my recent purchase from Big Al. I'm not easily bullied. I returned to my car and armed myself to the teeth. A pirate captain ready to seize the Spanish galleon just departing Panama for Cadiz, laden with Aztec and Incan treasure, and I climbed the stairs to my apartment ready to laugh about my misgivings and the surplus of a few Westinghouse watts.

The front door was locked, just as I had left it that morning, and the key fit smoothly and unimpeded. I slammed the door open, exactly as I remembered from the cowboy and gangster movies that wasted my childhood, catching the intruder behind it, while I rushed in and faced the other direction, covering both sides of the doorway. My finger on the trigger of my .38-caliber, while I called the name of my mother and my neighbor, Mrs. Linderman, my loved ones with keys to my apartment—drilling your mom or next door mate was not inscribed in the oath I took when I graduated medical school.

*Bang*, went the door, nobody behind it and no one to my right, when a big arm circled my neck, the other arm hitting my right hand, my gun dropping to the floor with a clatter. I slumped down as Mr. Big, whom I found out only later was not a hormonal giant, just a very big guy and my old street friend, standing adjacent to and not behind the slammed door, let go of my neck and retrieved the gun.

"Doc, it's about time you showed up." Big Guy laughed, my gun now in his possession. "We've been waiting a long time. Too long. You guys work too hard. You need a union, better hours and better pay. And there's nothing in the fridge. Nada. Zip. Zilch. Next time a little cream soda or Green River would be neighborly, and oh, I've got bad news for you, the Wonder Bread's spoiled—lots of little white spots all over it. Me and the boss gave it a pass."

Boss, my old baseball bat buddy, was apparently enjoying a recent promotion. Recovered from his infirmities, he was sitting comfortably on my wooden, folding kitchen chair currently stationed in the living room. His feet were jacked up on my faux Shaker-style coffee table with cruciform posts, one wooden leg replaced with stacked, outdated high school biology texts. The top of the table, battered from tabletop hockey tournaments, starred as the entertainment center of my used furniture collection and no one was allowed to rest their feet on it. Under different circumstances, I'd tell Mr. Baseball to obey visitor etiquette and at least remove his shoes.

The former minor leaguer was without his trademark Louisville Slugger. "Doc, let's go, we need to meet some fellows about business," was his only greeting.

"My friend," I said, "when you don't have your Babe Ruth model with you, it's serious isn't it?"

"Doc, let's go quietly. We're not like Tim. We can be quick and civilized, but only if you behave."

"You should know that Sergeant George Esposito and some of his policeman pals are around the house," I told the thugs. "They're somewhere close. Maybe you two should just quietly leave. There'll be no hard feelings, cross my heart,"—my right hand moved back and forth on my chest with my exclamation. "It'll be okay, don't worry. I'll tell them you were looking for the beauty salon, but made a wrong turn. But before I do anything, I have to go to the washroom and take a leak. It can't wait. I should've gone at the hospital, but I was in a hurry to get home."

The police threat didn't bother my friends, and I knew we weren't planning on rest stops. Big Guy, at first bemused, was now annoyed, as I turned my back on the two of them and quickly walked into my bedroom before they could respond, snapping the door behind me. No bullets or fists. They weren't anxious to waste me here.

"Doc, we've checked the windows, you can't go anywhere. Don't cause trouble for us. We can make life very unpleasant for you," Nikolai V yelled at me.

I pulled my second gun from my waistband under my coat, then moved to the right of the door in the darkened bedroom.

"Let me find some sheet music," I yelled back. "It'll make our trip seem shorter. I have 'Peg o' My Heart' for three way harmony somewhere around here."

Big Guy came bursting in, unhappy with the idea of me wasting their time and not being in his line of sight. On the other hand, he had dealt with me before, and what could I really do in my bedroom except start a pillow fight? The pistol, my former pistol, was rotating around his index finger, like he was a hyperactive child playing with a plastic ring toy. '*Big Guy,*' I wanted to tell him, '*stop playing with the gun that way. Remember what your mother said: "Handle those dangerous playthings carefully or you'll hurt yourself. You know what happened to one-eyed Ralphie.*" But Big Guy wouldn't have listened. He was that kind of kid. And he didn't need to be ready to shoot me. I was the weakling down the block.

It was his last mistake.

I shot him in the chest. The noise was deafening, reverberating around the room like von Trapp family yodels. There was nothing to absorb the sound. Maybe Sophie and I should have been quieter with our monkey business. The bullet hit something important. There was pain mixed with the surprise. The velocity of the shell stopped Big Guy in his tracks, but true soldier that he was, he raised his pistol, trying to right it, seeking me out in the darkness, and then I shot him again, and then for old time's sakes, I shot him once more as he slumped down, whispering for his mother.

"Asshole, I told you nottoshoothimhere, we need to get out of here fast." My minor league baseball friend burst into the room, angry, but unaware that it was me who was doing the enforcing.

"I also shot Mr. Baseball in the chest. The noise was in synch with Mrs. Linderman's banging on the wall. "Quiet in there, Doctor, I'm old and trying to get some sleep."

My second shot was off target, hitting my unhappy and now-trying-to-stand-up adversary in the leg. I didn't aim there, and the .38-caliber weapon felt heavy, like the weight of several cans of premium soup with hearty portions of meat. Tremors were developing in all of my extremities, and I could barely hold the thing upright. Mr. Baseball fell down; chest and thigh wounds were similar to a game-ending double play.

On the phone, Mrs. Esposito said, "I'm supposed to tell you that George is on his way. Don't leave the house. Lock yourself in the bathroom."

"Thanks, Mrs. Esposito, and have a nice night."

Locking myself in the bathroom sounded refreshing, with a long, hot-tub-bath, a bubble bath maybe, toy ships bobbing around me, my mother scrubbing my back, gently as only she could, while the bubbles started to cover my head and overflow onto the floor because I used the whole bottle of stuff instead of a capful as I was instructed.

I opened the front door again, not wanting damage there, as the sirens became closer. The Doppler effect was in place. It's a real fact, as I listened to the change in the sound waves being compressed as they sped toward me. My landlord was going to be pissed about the commotion. The police also didn't need to create further trouble by breaking the door down.

I let George and two of his uniformed friends in, pistols drawn, my hands up, no friendly-fire death for me. My gun was placed on the floor, easy to spot, sirens screaming in the background, as more protectors of citizens began to pile into my apartment, assuredly keeping Mrs. Linderman from her therapeutic sleep.

Nikolai V was still breathing, but no one was eager to call a city ambulance, while the task force searched my apartment, guns drawn, bulletproof vests snug tight over their uniforms.

"George, if you don't call an ambulance for my baseball buddy, I will," I said while I stood quietly in a corner, still with my hands over my head.

George picked up my gun, handkerchief in his hand, not wanting to sully the piece with his fingerprints, looking it over in disbelief, noting its newness, then stared at it again, finally barking into his walkie-talkie, requesting an ambulance.

"Doc, I can't believe it, two guns again. You're a marvel. Where's the one I sent you?"

I pointed to the dead big guy, still grasping the .38-caliber pistol that George had gifted me. The sergeant's grin parodied the enjoyment of viewing your first Road Runner cartoon or a glimpse of your newborn.

"Doc, the gun we gave you was special. We were planning on planting it on these bad guys, and here it's in the big guy's hand. His fingerprints will be all over it. That gun has killed at least two rival gangsters, possibly more, and just think, Doc, you're so great, we didn't even have to plant it on anyone. Now if only Mr. Baseball had been shot through the heart, we'd give you an A+. But it's okay, you still earn an A. Not bad," he said, the sergeant had no empathy for bad guys.

Baseball Guy was spitting at me. "Jesus, a doc with two guns, can you believe it? Doc, let's call it even, huh, and please don't visit me in the hospital, if I make it there, Godwilling. Where's the fucking ambulance?"

The evidence techs got there before the ambulance. I listened to Nikolai V's chest. His ribs were shattered at the entry wound, but he was aerating the lung out to the periphery. The bullet must have been deflected by his overgrown bones. The bleeding from the leg was ooze, no arterial pumping. Maybe he was going to make it.

The paramedics were pros. They paid no attention to me, starting IV fluids, a tourniquet around the thigh, and they gently carted Mr. Baseball away with police escort off to the County Hospital. I didn't let surprise register on my face, watching my old friend, the pimply-faced paramedic, capably handle the emergency. "Good job," I told him. I prayed for the opportunity to sit down with him, to offer acne treatment gratis, and to talk things over cordially. The combination of an orally administered, low-dose, tetracycline antibiotic, plus a cleansing ointment applied several times daily, would vitalize his personality. Collecting disability pay and still working for a living was all right in my world, and I'm a forgiving kind of guy, as I gave him the thumbs-up. I'd notify Jane the next day.

"Mr. Minor Leaguer and friend were going to kill you, you know," George spoke. "They were told to get even for Tim."

"George, that was big-time, why didn't you tell me about their whereabouts tonight and how did they tie me in with Tim's murder?"

I knew the answers, but I wasn't going to discuss them with George.

I needed to sit down. It was like scrubbing in on an all-day Whipple procedure. Intravenous fluids would help, and if I could lay my head down for a little while, I'd be myself again.

"We were following these guys, but I thought they were going home for the night and my guys needed some beers and we had to catch up on the sports. But you didn't need our help." George placed his hand on my shoulder in admiration, and became surprised by my shudder of revulsion.

"George, don't touch me," I told him. "You gave me a gun with that history and left me this exposed! Take my statement or whatever you need, and then I have to call Stan Glicke. I want a lawyer with me and then we're history. Don't ever mention the Tomczak thing again unless it comes with a subpoena. Cancel the backyard swimming parties and forget the hot dogs and bratwursts and me joining the all-American neighbors slumming at your house."

The crowd massed in front of my quiet neighborhood abode, the television trucks, the reporters pushing their microphones in our faces. Mrs. Linderman, now fully awake and dressed in holiday finery, nicely asked if I was okay, while I muttered to her and to everyone else who asked, "*No comment.*"

George and his captain proudly expounded about the wheels of justice. Two criminals bent on revenge were shot by the hero doctor. The gurney with a body bag stretched to its limit, requiring eight hands to carry down the stairs, was showered with appreciative murmurs from the crowd as they viewed the remains of someone the size of Frankenstein plus Igor. Children, all of whom should have been asleep at this hour, were being lifted on shoulders to view the spectacle of a body bag—a dispirited hero—me, strutting police, and Mrs. Linderman sashaying around, surprisingly light on her feet for this occasion, her walker nowhere in sight, permed blue hair freshly sprayed tight for the cameras, mischief glowing from her as she sang: "*That's my neighbor, he's a podiatrist.*"

Now she's standing in front of the television camera expounding skillfully for the network viewers: "You know he's a hero. Just look at him. Strong and manly, and he's such a considerate neighbor. Sometimes when one of his girlfriends is over—he's single by the way—but don't get excited girls, I saw him first. And his accordion-playing is heavenly. I get up and dance to it, but don't tell him that because I've complained about the noise."

*"The hero doctor apparently turned the table on the two gangsters waiting for him in his apartment, here on Damen Avenue, normally a quiet street in a quiet part of the city. The details aren't clear, but one of the presumed gangsters has been shot dead. The police haven't provided the name of the deceased. The other gangster was shot in the chest and has been taken to County Hospital. This was the doctor recently caught up in a drug deal gone bad, the recipient of a beating, reported first by our news team. More details to follow, as soon as they become available. This is Mary Julienne Tinker reporting for Channel Two News."*

# SIX

The coincidences of life follow a recognizable rhythm. I attended my last anger management class the next morning held in the hospital conference room down the hall from the chief's office. Sweet rolls and coffee, but no knives or forks for obvious reasons. The reception for the "doctor gunman" pictured in the evening television news and morning newspapers was muted. Dr. Gershon needed only a moment to compose her thoughts after welcoming me, pleased that I was intact, and asked if I was able to demonstrate restraint in my activities of the previous night.

"Yes, Dr. Gershon, I shot the second bad guy only twice, thanks to your wisdom," the words spoken as I sat down, breaking the ice, because I received hugs and kisses from the women with anger problems and firm handshakes from the male reprobates.

"That was amazing what happened to you," was the best that I could receive from the good Dr. Gershon, but her hug and concern were appreciated. "Sleepless nights and relentless anxiety are sure to follow the violence," she said and suggested further counseling. I agreed.

Next up was the chief. Mrs. Gail was pleased to see me. She had been concerned about the mechanics of my taking medical call while receiving protective custody. High heels clomped the familiar pathway to the chief's office, but no words, just a knock on the chief's door and the usual thumb pointed my way.

"Chief, my criminal-related activities are over," I said, my first words to him. I toed the new party line set in motion by Sergeant Esposito. "I was a witness to a drug deal and the two gangsters wanted to ensure my silence and they screwed up. I was lucky, having been pre-warned by the hardworking police." I didn't mention Tim or Betty.

The chief could smell a mistruth, but was pleased that I was back and not hurt. The flurry of news, the reporters beseeching Mrs. Gail, demanding sketches of my daily life—"Doctor by Day, Avenger at Night"—would hopefully end soon.

"We're doctors all the time," the chief told me. "That doesn't leave much time for other activities. I know you'll remember that. You and Howard are able to provide some respite from the grind with your music and crazy antics, but this police involvement is too much." He shook his head. "This is all new to me. At morning report, tell everybody about the diagnostic coup with the VIP banker. I know Manny Cohen and the chest surgeon didn't make the diagnosis. You did. Dr. Brown telephoned me earlier to sing your praises before telling me you routinely barge into his office without waiting for an invitation and that must stop."

Mrs. B slid off her stool and poured a cup, well, a half a cup of coffee for me, even before I got near the coffee line. "My hero," a hug, and then, I didn't know what more to expect, another hug or a headlock as she handed me the coffee, *gratis*, except for the on-call coupons that she was willing to accept all of a sudden.

"Thank you, Mrs. B, I'll owe you more coupons. I get new ones this week." And I returned her embrace. A meaningful one, since the events of yesterday were affecting my mind and body with too much epinephrine, serotonin, and dopamine combined in unusual portions and bathing my brain cells while playing with my mood.

Estelle joined me for coffee, although she had to pay for the privilege of drinking the dark stuff. "You're my champion, and you're invited to my wedding in spite of what Fineglass says about you." She offered me her hand to be kissed—a heavenly blend of sweet roll and woman goodness.

"Thanks Estelle, and thanks for inviting me to your wedding. I'm honored. "Estelle, do you know Carl Sandburg?"

"What floor is he on?" she asked.

"He wrote: *People like us/us two/we own the moon*."

My poetry recitation elicited a smile that quickly vanished when I continued.

"I have the perfect gift for your wedding night, and now I'll be able to bring it to you in person on that soon-to-arrive magical day. Mail can't express my deep-felt thoughts about your nuptials. When the excitement of the ceremony and the party winds down and your lovely self has slipped into your brand-new, slinky black negligee, and your perfume has been spotted in wonderful places, although to be honest with you Estelle, you don't need additional perfume, then deliver the gift to Fineglass.

"Believe me," I spoke to my beauty, "I've thought hard about selecting an offering that will please Fineglass and provide something that will keep him busy in a productive sort of way. Good for you, good for his patients, good for him, it's a gift trifecta," I continued. "*The Official Crossword Puzzle Book for Surgeons*, complete with crayons, different colors no less, but each very bright, and wouldn't you know, and it's his good fortune, they're the extra thick ones, easy to grasp, even for people with stubby fingers. And the simple instructions are printed in large type and the puzzles themselves have no words longer than four letters. This will excite him big time."

"You've just been relegated to the children's table," Estelle responded to my wondrous gift description, her chair falling over backward as she abruptly exited.

"I haven't seen Nurse Sophie in a long time, and Dr. Estelle surely left quickly," Mrs. B told me, walking over and sitting next to me, leaving the fallen chair for someone else to remedy. "Beautiful women like us desire a quiet type of person. Contemplative, even. You know what that word means, don't you, Doctor? Richer also, of course, and good dancers, too, just a few suggestions you might consider because you look lonely, what with yet another lovely woman leaving your table in a huff."

"Thank you for the advice, Mrs. B. I need all the help you can offer. And thanks for the coffee, it's delicious today," I was lying to her without even thinking about it. But she didn't hear me, because someone in line was whining about the status of the bananas: "Too brown, too soft," lifting each of them up for us to see, while Mrs. B shouted back—"I saw that! Once you've touched them they're yours," then shaking her head and mumbling to herself, "Get a load of that sorry doofus."

Chuck, the chief resident, stopped by, carrying a handful of sugar packets and stirrers snatched from the cafeteria. "Why are you having coffee here and not at the chief's office?" he asked.

"Because I wasn't invited, Mr. Chief Resident, and don't worry about pilfering the sugar. I'll have Mrs. B place it on my bill." For someone so smart, why did that comment pass right over his head?

Finally, Howard joined me. "You weren't invited to the chief's office either?" I asked him.

"I'd rather be here with you good buddy," he told me, while he yelled over to Mrs. B. Her name was now permanently "Mrs. B" and she answered reliably to that moniker: "Some draft ale for my friend and for me also, *por favor*." In return, he received the finger from our lovely Mrs. B, displayed in front of the many people who were milling around. Mrs. B not caring at all what they thought. People who ate at her establishment were provincial. The big-time hospital administrators never dined there, always ordering out, Chinese, or deli plates, or pizza, or Mr. Beef. You could tell what day of the week it was by which delivery truck was sitting outside the president's office. So who of importance would ever see Mrs. B flash the finger at the two resident doctors?

"Howard, I need some antidepressants. Will they work on a gunman like me, a combination of Mr. Crack Shot and Mr. Lonely? Phil's in Florida visiting Sophie. I miss her. I've completed anger management classes without accomplishing a thing. I'm sure Dr. Gershon thinks I'm hopeless. When I dream about being featured in the newspapers, as I was yesterday and today, I assumed it would be for my medical discoveries. Our picture, you and me, microphone in hand, graciously thanking our teachers and the 'little people' for Nobel Prize-type stuff. Not me plastered on the front cover for wasting people. No coffee or single-malt Scotch with the chief, and Estelle is really marrying Dr. Manslaughter, the doctor with no detectable skills or personality."

# SEVEN

Next morning I met with Stan, now my official lawyer, with lawyer-client privileges. The nominal fee was paid with a check, and I could tell him about the source of the guns and the happenings of the night involving the thugs and George. He listened quietly and intently, taking a few written notes, being nonjudgmental, with an occasional head nod and we were ready to meet the district attorney and his staff.

I provided another official statement, identical to the one I had given the night of the killing. The gun found in Mr. Big Guy's hand had been used in several mob-type killings. So Big Guy must have been involved. George ordered me not to mention that the police had provided the armament. The assistant DA, the intense-looking blond woman who couldn't sit still chimed in: "Boss,"—she was talking to Mr. DA—"isn't it unusual for these guys to keep the weapons with them and use them more than once? Don't they toss them after a single use?"

"I don't think this thug was so smart. He was missing the gray, so to speak," countered our DA.

It's so easy to estimate the IQ of the deceased.

"Thanks to this quick-thinking doctor we've solved several murders and the wrongdoers have been punished," he continued.

We nodded in agreement, even though Mr. DA had lost my vote in the upcoming general election. I would have liked to have told them that most likely it was George Esposito who gave my baseball bat-swinging friend the orders to come after me. Nikolai V or Big Guy didn't initiate the ambush. But Mr. Photogenic DA just shook his head, his gelled hair tight with Brylcreem, and smiled in wonderment when I brought up Mr. Baseball's intelligence.

I was to be nominated for official civilian hero. The DA's handshake was firm and his smile sincere. He wasn't going to miss my vote. Nobody thought there would be recriminations. The two bad guys were out of action, one of course being dead. They had been aligned with Tim Schmidt, also recently deceased, and if there was a turf war, I had nothing to do with it. We smiled again.

Stan and I talked over a beer and shrimp cocktail at his favorite bar. We thought our voting for anyone running against the DA was our civic duty. I declined Stan's offer for a weekend in the Caribbean that included sun, warmth, girls, rum and Coke, plural on all items, while I wrote two prescriptions for antibiotics, insisting that one be used by him.

"We'll see," he said, smiling and shaking his head no ever so slightly. We switched to Bombay Sapphire martinis over ice with just a twist of lemon peel, as we both needed to taste nirvana. For Stan, it was for his trip and his fantasies, and for me it was for freedom from jail and guilt.

# EIGHT

Howard and I traveled to the university. Although the academic year didn't start for several more months, their Department of Medicine sponsored a lunch for incoming fellows. Howard would be a first-year trainee in gastroenterology—a highly sought-after position. His good looks and brains and not necessarily his friendship with me had enriched his competitive position. His parents' donation toward the new research unit also might have boosted his application, but that was speculation on my part.

After lunch, we split up. I went to the inpatient hematology floor to meet Dr. Mollman. A new life was starting for me—the quiet and sincere me using my hard-earned medical skills to their fullest extent. Mother, Harry, and my late departed father would be proud, and the chief also, and Mrs. Gail, and everyone else in my life. Plus, I would have a good time. And I had just sent Sophie an invitation to attend the end-of-the-year graduation party for the IntMed 3s.

While I was standing at the nurses' desk waiting for Dr. Mollman, the head nurse pulled my arm toward her and pleaded, "Doctor, please come quick and help me with the patient in 603B." Her look of concern was reason enough for me to peek in on the lady, who was gasping for air, and if there was a heartbeat, I couldn't detect it with my ear to her chest.

"Call your arrest code, stat," I ordered and started closed-chest massage. "Is there an ECG monitor on the floor? If so, please get it, right after you dial your code." I pushed the nurse to the telephone between chest compressions. I could now feel a carotid pulse, feeble and too quick. Maybe this was going to be a treatable arrhythmia.

The code team rushed in, the medical resident, a clone of me, in charge and asking for information about the patient. When I didn't even know why the patient was hospitalized, he asked me who the hell I was and suggested I step aside. I was glad to comply, and his team took over. The ECG monitor revealed a supraventricular tachycardia, correctly diagnosed by this team. They drew blood, started IV fluids, and attached a blood pressure monitor. "Start a pressor and procainamide," they ordered. I agreed, but they didn't consult with me.

The nurse was gracious enough to thank me, and I left the patient in good hands. I was impressed. The code resident had danced around just like I did.

Dr. Mollman wasn't so pleased. "Where've you been, Dr. Ted? I've been here for ten minutes standing around waiting for you. You come with such a reputation for screwing off, and here you're late for our first meeting." He wasn't that pissed, just making sure I knew his ground rules. "Doctor," he said, offering wisdom, "misdeeds, jokes, tardiness, sex, all last only minutes—being a doctor takes a lifetime."

"Thanks, Dr. Mollman, sorry to be late, it won't happen again. Thanks for being patient with me, and I understand what you're saying." We made rounds. Mixed in with his showing off his clinical skills, we talked about research goals. We got along fine.

The hematology people had a show-and-tell party. Their research covered a wide spectrum. Sitting in tight individual groups, there were the oncologists, the leukemia people with Dr. Mollman, the blood clotting clique, and the immunology team, with Dr. Brennan and Sarah. I joined the latter. Apparently this was a day for impressing one another. I wasn't sure I was a prize, but everyone said hello. Most likely, they were fearful I'd shoot out their tires if they didn't flash a friendly face. The abundance of talent reinforced my decision about training in their program.

The joy ended quickly, as it so often does in medicine. My beeper went bonkers the moment I stepped back into the hospital. Gertrude, the page operator, said I was needed on the oncology floor. A page about anything there was bad news.

"I'm not on call for Oncology," I yelled at Gertrude. After my almost three years here, we had nary a kind word for one another.

"Doctor, don't scream at the operator. I'm just reading what was handed to me. It says you're to see a Professor Bernstein in room 407 per order of Dr. Rhoban. Would you like me to tell Dr. Rhoban and the professor that the message was delivered to you and you're not coming?"

"That's not necessary, Gertrude, and thanks for the kindness."

I could scream and hang up in anger, but the battle was too one-sided. Combativeness was the *lingua franca* of the page operators, and anonymous messages delivered to me from her colleagues in the middle of the night kept me in line.

The door to 407 was open. All the rooms on the cancer floor were the same: small, dimly lit, and painted blue. Blue was the color deemed by some wizard to improve the morale of the dying. It was noisy. The nurses frowned on you closing the door, keeping an eye on you as they patrolled the corridor, their voices loud, their medicine carts squeaky.

I knocked on the inner wall with no response. The professor was sleeping. Intravenous fluid hung overhead, dripping monotonously into his arm. The label on the bottle listed no medications, just fluid, most likely for hydration. He was thin, his skin pale and flabby, the hospital gown too large, its folds doubled over on his chest, so unlike the beauty of his crisp tailored suits and starched shirts. A chair had been placed next to the head of the bed. I sat down and touched his cheek, softly calling his name.

Music softened the hospital clamor. Faure's "Pavane" serenaded from a portable radio placed near the foot of the bed. Everyone knows the "Pavane," but it should have been the "Requiem" playing.

He awakened gently. His dream must have been peaceful, and he propped himself up to a sitting position, waving away my attempt to help.

"So good to see you, Doctor," he said, his voice hoarse. "Just pour some water for me." He pointed to the pitcher on the other side of the bed. The water was cold; moisture beaded on the outside of the clear plastic cup holding a tall paper straw bent at an obtuse angle.

The professor let me hold the cup for him as he struggled to sit more upright, his lips parched and stiff. His mouth had difficulty circling the straw. He was thirsty and the liquid made a gurgling sound when he swallowed.

"I won't beat around the bush, my Polish friend." His voice was stronger and higher-pitched after drinking the water. "The doctors tell me that the lymphoma cells somehow have learned to resist the poisons they've given me. They're all very kind, the doctors, acting as if they are surprised by the developments, patting me on my back and making clucking noises in sympathy. Just between us, my friend, their noise and their sad looks have become obscene. You know, I've already undergone a course of brain radiation." With that he stopped, his throat catching. The enormity of a person of his intellect receiving palliative treatment that killed brain cells was not lost on either of us.

I stayed silent. I resisted joining the fraternity of doctors clucking in disappointment and nodding their heads up and down like cockatoos on perches.

"They have some experimental medicine they want to try. The experts claim it will make me only a little sick. A 'little sick,' of course, is doctor pabulum for constant retching. Well, you know that."

The professor had become exhausted with his speech, holding his palm up for a time-out. "You know I was teaching until ten days ago.

"Doctor," he said, his eyes misting as they searched mine. "Do you think you can help me with a prescription or injection of something to take home so I can meet my maker? I need your help. And I appreciate the goodness and reason that you possess."

"Sure, sure," I said, first looking toward the door and then the window, trying to stay poised. "I remember." His words caught me off-guard. I wanted to say no, but the Professor had been my teacher, a gift-giver, a giant in medicine, and I couldn't turn away from him in his time of need.

"Dr. Rhoban shook his head when I asked him for assistance. 'There are many other treatment options to try,' he told me, 'and new ones are being developed every day,' and then he patted me on the back, his head moving north and south. His parting words were: 'Hang tough, Professor, the battle has just started, and together we'll manage.'"

# NINE

If you think your life unwinds too quickly, spend a year or three as a medical resident. Nighttime call, holiday duties, a pending qualifying examination—time passes faster than Chicago's Indian summer. My turnaround jump shot had turned to shit, and my music appreciation bordered on a depressing C-. It didn't help that my new car radio had been stolen from the doctors' parking lot. Of all the cars to steal from, Mercedes parked everywhere, and Cadillacs too numerous to count, but to be fair, their car locks and alarms were functional.

So many people to say goodbye to, starting at the subbasement, shaking hands with the morgue guys, and then a hug, a long one, considerably embarrassing Dr. Wendle, one of the good people residing on earth. My goodbye rounds included the radiologists. They were a good sort, offering stock market tips and real estate investment advice along with their diagnostic pearls.

Nurses and technicians from the entire medical center received cards from Howard and me, reminding them how we had provided fun, merriment, sensual thoughts, literary advice, and music suggestions during the last three years. I'm sure they were appreciative and were going to miss us, because our car windows remained egg-free.

My physical diagnosis students needed special attention. They were heading into their third year of medical school with the scary rotations—delivering babies, attending sick children, scrubbing in with the surgeons, many of whom were laden with personality disorders manifested by violence, or at a minimum, foul language directed at the students' perceived shortcomings, depicting them as garbage or poop or something of that ilk.

Sharon was interested in internal medicine. Bright, personable, and facile with medical procedures, she was able to approach veins with confidence. I witnessed her taking a streptococci throat culture without swiping nasal droppings or removing plaque etched onto canine teeth. I suggested several programs that were a good fit and congratulated her on her choice of pathways. Clinical rotations with top-notch teachers such as the chief and Herb Rhoban would hone her skills.

Ron had become interested in psychiatry. I don't think it was because he hoped to help me tackle some of my problems, and it wasn't because of any ineptitude in the physical aspects of medicine. He was good with his hands and mind. It turned out that quiet, bespectacled Ron liked talking to people, delving into their inner workings. Of course, we all did, especially when the patients were young and of the opposite gender.

Bert and Phyllis's ambitions were unformed. They were still lingering in the background, trying to assess life, a little overwhelmed with the scope of a profession that offered so many options and opportunities. They would be good doctors. Bert's interest in surgery wavered. He liked the drama of the OR, but the hours were grueling. Phyllis matured at every session, newfound confidence unfolding with every new patient; she stood straighter, offered well-timed probing questions, and even an occasional comfortable laugh. It was my good fortune that all four of my students had promise and a sense of fun. The latter would help them stay on an even keel through the ordeal of medical training.

We lunched together on their last day. Mrs. B allowed me to reserve a table in the rear of the cafeteria usually reserved for the comatose. One of the serving people waited on us, as if we were dining in a classy restaurant. She came in and assisted me for a few bucks on her day off. The sign on the table read, PRIVATE PARTY RESERVED and linen napkins and metal utensils made us feel important while we shooed our colleagues away.

The special meal was tomato soup, fresh from the Campbell's can, salad served cold with green onions and cucumbers, Kraft Italian dressing placed in fringed paper cups on the side, and spaghetti with meat sauce. Mrs. B surprised us with her homemade rice pudding, carefully ladling out servings, even for me, narrating the history of her family's favorite dessert passed down through generations. It went especially well with chamomile tea with lemon, she told all of us, staring unblinkingly at me during her monologue.

# TEN

The professor's lymphoma responded to the new treatment. That's what usually happened. It was satisfying to watch the lymph nodes melt away. The doctors were pleased with their plan. Everyone was filled with hope. Of course, it was temporary.

Roger Maris hit sixty-one homers, breaking Babe Ruth's thirty-four-year-old record; the Russians detonated Tsar Bomba, 1,400 times more powerful than the bombs dropped on Japan; the British left Kuwait forever; Hurricane Hattie devastated Belize City. There was not much room in the newspaper or television news for a teacher and innovator and godsend for many, who took his own life before the lymphoma could.

*Primum non nocere* is Latin for "first do no harm." It's beat into us repeatedly from the first day of medical school. It's our fundamental principle. One would think I would have learned it. My prescription for one-hundred morphine tablets dispensed in a plastic vial from the hospital pharmacy, one tablet every four hours as needed for pain, now empty, had been found at the professor's bedside.

From time to time, I awaken with palpitations. My dream, etched in granite, as if trying to catch trains failing to stop for me, or wandering aimlessly through pitch-black hospital corridors leading nowhere, isn't nasty enough, the woman with pedunculated skin lesions sits hunched over in a tiny examining room, chanting "*primum non nocere*" shedding tears the size of hail falling in early spring storm. Thicker than a fist they bounce high off the floor and engulf me as if I'm trapped under a Swiss avalanche. I cry out for help, but my words are silent.

# ELEVEN

Weddings trump funerals. Estelle and Fineglass were married in a North Side temple, standing under a canopy called a *chuppah* sheltering a community of people: the bride and groom, the rabbi, and just about everyone else of blood ancestry, all of whom were permanently slumped over in an acute angle of fatigue. The Hebrew intonations, the bride walking around the groom seven times, as Joshua circled the walls of Jericho, the stomping of the wine goblet, the *Mazel Tovs*, the Bach and Pachelbel borrowed from a rival religion, the rabbi's silly jokes, the officious introduction of Dr. and Dr. Fineglass, as if two doctors never marry—it was wonderful.

The downtown hotel reception was fancy, but not of the grandeur of the future Jane and Howard nuptials. The newly married couple hired their own band, the musicians a year or so away from shaving. Howard and I would patiently wait for the creative moment before kidnapping the entertainment. Duke Ellington once said: "You can say anything you want on the trombone, but you gotta be careful with words." That wouldn't work for us. We would disrupt this place with both music and words.

I came alone. Sophie couldn't get away, a last-moment thing. "Is Phil visiting you or was it what we talked about in Florida?" I asked. There was no reply. Sandra from Craig Tollen, the aortic aneurysm, VIP banker, only laughed, but laughed pleasantly, when declining my invitation. Sarah and Amy weren't available.

My table card had a three-digit number. Fineglass did have a sense of humor. Not sitting with Jane and Howard and to bond with the nieces and nephews and other children was okay with me, but the tiny folding chairs created lower lumbar spine discomfort. On the other hand, special party favors were present at this table, along with neat conical hats usually gifted at birthday gatherings, the kind worn point up, court jester-like, with the rubber band holding it in place and cutting deep into your chin. But good fortune struck. Dr. Gershon poked my arm—"The mister was called away on business and couldn't attend. Sit with me, Ted," she said. "I know you enjoy dancing."

"No, I don't like to dance, good Doctor, and I'll need assistance selecting the proper eating utensils, separating bread and salad plates, and then there's always asparagus tips trapped between my front teeth, and yes, I'd very much like to be your tablemate. Thank you."

There was a paucity of eligible young men standing around, plus Dr. Gershon had already asked me to be her guest, so there was no turning back. I kissed the back of her warm hand, and admired her black shift. Her bare shoulders were loosely covered with a near-transparent, black-laced scarf; her hair, decorously piled up and tinted pitch-black competed with her dress for attention. She took a deep breath and offered me a smile. Psychiatrists were cool and especially so at weddings. They understood better than anyone the dynamics between warring families, and they were the only doctors attending the ceremony and reception not expected to assist at the fainting or emesis or chest pain disasters.

Psychiatrist and patient, we made our rounds of the tables, outwardly a success story, but both of us aware of my shortcomings. Even years of psychotherapy rarely changed the inner you. On the other hand, I wasn't in jail or hospitalized in a psychiatric ward, and all of my troubles were forgotten this night, as we toasted the happiness of Fineglass and Estelle.

The pall as we approached Table Four was similar to the reception afforded the sailing ships hoisting the yellow fever flag when entering a tropical harbor, while we joined the chief and his wife, Dr. and Mrs. Rhoban, Wendy and Naomi, and the hospital president and his missus—our seats strategically placed between the chief and the hospital president.

Circling the table, I made my rounds, shaking hands with the tuxedoed VIPs and bussing the elegant women. How fascinating it would be for the latter when they regaled their canasta and book club cronies about sharing the table with the handsome young doctor, the same one who was marched through the hospital in handcuffs by city policemen. The very same doctor who shot two hoodlums, killing one of them!

"You remember all that don't you, Doreen?" they'd say. "It was pictured in all the newspapers. And yet he seemed like a normal-appearing person, polite, ate dinner with a fork and knife. Yes, they actually let him have the latter, and there was no drooling or spittle, and I looked for it, surreptitiously of course, because as you know, they can become violent quicker than a mother grizzly."

It was a many course dinner, interrupted by speeches and blessings and dancing. Edith would look at me, point to the dance floor, and I would shake my head, just a nod, almost imperceptible, because I was too busy socializing with contemporaries making pilgrimages to our table and savoring the satisfying pregnant pauses that occurred after the visitors sized up the Table Four pairings. The hospital president and Dr. Ted!

I will attempt to arrange these unconventional table assignments for future parties. The clanking of our wine and champagne glasses, the eye contact and smiles welcomed the supplicants. And the bigwigs at Table Four set a fine example for the young doctors with their facile introductions and exemplary table manners.

I waved to Mrs. Gail at Table Nineteen, bragging about my recent ascension in this world by holding up four fingers and pointing to my surroundings. Jealousy printed boldly on her face. You might not be able to anticipate your successes, but when they arrive, be sure to notify everyone.

Fineglass was a handsome groom with his well-fitting tuxedo; his surgeon's hands were prominently displayed for the relatives. If I heard, "*It's a wonderful match*," one more time, I'd puke on the floral centerpiece. That would lessen the jockeying over who would take it home.

Estelle and Fineglass visited each table, collecting envelopes, thin with certified checks, or thick with large-denomination currency thrust at them by family members. They posed next to the multi-tiered wedding cake, turning red-eyed with camera flashes. Two plastic figures were featured on the top of the pastry, a tuxedoed doctor sporting a Groucho Marx mustache and holding a stethoscope and otoscope, and the other—heavy-breasted and matronly appearing, staring adoringly at her new spouse—misogyny prospered even at weddings between doctors.

The photographer made it to each table. The several with me and the chief, each smiling for the camera, not necessarily toward one another, would be priceless.

"Would you like to dance?" I asked my psychiatrist.

"You're slow, but like the proverbial tortoise you eventually get there. Yes, I would," she said.

Every band has the same routine. First the slow stuff, the foxtrot or waltz, allowing conversation, romance not far away from your thoughts, and then something faster, a jitterbug, the twist, the latter a new and devilish delight that offered no respite for the exhausted. Then a faster dance—who knew what the music was—only Howard and Jane, the bride and groom, and my psychiatrist and I were left showcasing the quick steps.

Howard and I excused ourselves from our partners, took the bride's hands, edging out the surgeon, and the three of us shook our pelvises and threw our arms over our heads. Too sensual for the young bandleader, who switched into the Hora, as we kicked up our legs to the words of "*Hava Nagila*"— and all of the guests joined us, forming intertwining lines—Dr. Gershon and I reuniting, the two of us performing the steps and still able to laugh.

"Here it comes." The invitees poked their dates in the ribs as Howard and I bullied our way to the stage, followed by silence broken only by the clatter of spoons and knives settling into dinner plates and soup bowls. Nudging the sixteen-year-old bandleader off the soprano side of the bench, Howard and I commandeered the piano. Howard, tuxedoed, in charge, announced the playbill: "A song for Estelle and Fineglass, but especially for the latter, played from our hearts for the wonderful and beautiful newlyweds."

"Shrimp Boats" was a popular piece, indeed a number-one song in *Your Hit Parade* for weeks, but it was our creative libretto that made it especially brilliant.

*The shrimp guy is a-comin'*

With one hand pounding the piano, the other following Fineglass around, unable to escape our attention, although he tried, we chanted, "shrimp, shrimp, shrimp." The younger attendees, knowing the groom full well, also shifted into party mode, riffing along and pointing at Fineglass.

Oh, the joy of singing popular tunes that become louder at each reprise; fun, it was a lot of fun for everyone, save for one person. No make it two, Estelle didn't appear happy.

Our hands raised, the silence accentuating the recent chaos, and Howard and I continued, but no more tasteless words about limited intelligence or size, or singing our new composition entitled "Ambisinister," also known as "Clumsy with Both Hands." That would await another occasion.

We sang "Serenade of the Bells."

In that song, the parents of the lovers made only one condition to their marriage.

*That the Mission Bells had to ring.*

But—and that was a very big but—because:

*Everyone knew the bells were broken.*
*And hadn't sounded for a long, long time.*

Well, you can guess what happened.

*One night the village was astounded*
*For the bells began to chime!*

Because, you see, in the lovers' hearts a true love dwelled.

*They will ring in all their glory*
*That's the serenade of the bells.*

I stood up, facing the celebrants, and belted out the *ding-dongs*, while Howard tinkled the piano as only he could, the guests drowning in tears.

Dr. Gershon, now Edith, gave me a hug. "I was prepared for the worst after your first act, planning on sending you back to Table 151, but it's okay, you may continue to sit here."

"Maybe my days of therapy have been helpful, thank you," I told her.

The other Table Four guests remained silent. There exists among older people an uncertainty about what comprises good taste.

Every wedding party has a time set aside for the geriatric crowd before the real fun begins. Slow songs in bunches that we said "*ooh*" and "*aah*" about, while Estelle and Fineglass were passed around like newborns at a christening. Enough dancing so the over fifty crowd could go home tired and happy and leave the authentic celebrating, fortified with bottles of champagne hidden under the tables, for the youngsters.

"Thanks for the sweet song, Ted," Estelle murmured to me, holding up extraordinarily well at her own wedding and already willing to forgive me for our first opus.

"Howard and I asked Fineglass to join us in the entertainment," I said. "A guy trio thing, but he couldn't remember the words to the 'Alphabet Song.'" Estelle gracefully pirouetted away, only a trace of disgust settling on her lovely face.

Edith and I sipped coffee at the empty table after our dancing, our eyes grading the dancing couples. Wendy and Naomi, products of ballroom instruction, showed off their precisely timed turns, separating and returning in step and in rhythm. The Arthur Murray Dance Studio fees were well-earned.

"Ted, you're fun and clever." I received a nudge from my psychiatrist. "Thanks for sitting with me. You're good company for being both a psychoneurotic and deep-seated sociopath. The latter adds that extra edge of excitement that many people crave. And weddings are so romantic, look at Grandma and Grandpa Fineglass, over there, holding hands, their joy is palpable, and that lovely Department of Psychiatry nurse dancing with, oh, never mind, that's Mr. Gail.

"I'm staying at this hotel tonight," my psychiatrist continued, no change in voice or rhythm. "Mr. Gershon won't join me until tomorrow. I have a magnificent view of the lake, but you have to stand on a chair and angle it just right to see the gorgeous blue water merging with the sky. I need someone to steady my legs—the chair's kind of wobbly. How much help can I be with your counseling if I fall through the window? You'll need to hold me here," she said, placing my palm on her waist, shielded by the table and white linen tablecloth, her warm hand remaining on top of mine.

"Here's the key with the room number. You take the north elevator."

I made no unusual noises as I nonchalantly slurped the coffee, now too cold for pleasure. Seduction provided warmth.

"I also enjoy scenic views," I said, although her offer didn't seem to be a discussion, more like travel directions. "A late-night pillow fight is just the exercise that would do us both good after all this food," I added.

We parted, hands lightly touching, assignation in place. If this was how it's played at psychiatry conventions, I was entering the wrong specialty. It was probably too late in the evening for pirate costumes or Count Dracula capes.

I joined Howard and Jane, smug in my secret, while my psychiatrist and soon-to-be lover, graciously made her exit, a kind word for everyone, air-kisses here and there, saving her sweet lips for me.

# TWELVE

The city is beautiful at 4 a.m. The streetlights speckled my automobile with shades of pearl, as I rolled toward home. The stillness belied the energy that erupts at dawn. Carl Sandburg hit it on the head—at daybreak we would become the *Stormy, husky, brawling, City of the Big Shoulders*." But never quoted in the tourist brochures was the remainder of his creativity that adopted me: *And they tell me you are crooked and I answer/Yes, it is true I have seen the gunmen kill and go free to kill again.*

The second wind that's ours in the late evening and early morning was a prerequisite for medical training. We lie down for fifteen or twenty minutes, close our eyes, empty our brains, and find sleep. The dry, bitter grunge coating our mouths when we awakened provided the telltale sign that we had entered deep slumber. We were refreshed, capable of thinking and making decisions again. It's a gift. The crankiness showed up later.

Alert and at peace after the wedding and the passionate lovemaking with my dear psychiatrist, I was filled with buoyant energy, while I continued to drive around the block in spite of several inviting parking spaces.

History has a habit of repeating itself, or as George Santayana aptly proclaimed: "Those who cannot remember the past are condemned to repeat it." The seventy-five watt glow, the middle of the three way illumination left burning in the dormer window, was dark. It created a Pavlovian effect. The speed of light is overwhelmingly fast for human lives spent at puny walking paces or driving at the city's official speed limit of 25 miles per hour—and my thoughts switched from romance to Einstonian physics, because the lack of light, darkness, also travels fast.

Things happen of course. Light bulbs burn out all of the time, on a daily basis even. You can't travel through life spooked by faulty Westinghouse or G.E. three-way light bulbs and curse the darkness. Even Thomas Alva Edison had off-days.

I needed another pistol to bolster my bravery. Maybe I should awaken Mrs. Linderman and borrow her custom-handled Smith & Wesson. But I gave in to common sense. I found my favorite telephone booth, down the block, open and inviting, braved the cool drizzle, and called my sergeant. He'd said to call him anytime. Not that I trusted him, but who else could I telephone at this time of night.

I left the phone number on his beeper, resting my head on the closed hinged door, the sudden change in my mood contrasting with blissful pictures of my mind doctor. The return ring, prompt and loud in the subdued night, was as quick as the return of the luminosity glowing from my apartment window. Light and electricity travel at the same speed.

The sergeant should have had a flashlight, but then again even if he did, using the telephone in my apartment wasn't easy. Hard to locate, the phone was buried under textbooks and patient charts. Turning on a light would be a necessity.

"Ted, one moment." Recognizing my hello, he asked me to hold, while I heard his footsteps, and my apartment turned dark again.

"George, the light was off in my apartment; it should be on. I'm worried there's someone in there. I drove back to the hospital to page you," I said. "Can you or someone meet me in front so we can enter together?"

"Can do, Doc," he said. "Meet me in ten or fifteen minutes, I'm not far away. You did the right thing by paging me."

I waited a few minutes, and sure enough, the sergeant appeared at the front door, alone and not dressed for the chilliness and drizzle of the early morning, putting on his gloves one finger at a time.

"*No thanks, George*," I said to myself and headed back to my car. My good friend, the sergeant, had nothing pleasant in store for me. Waiting for me in the cold and damp, while I drove to the hospital, would be his reward.

Frank, the nighttime hospital security guard, nodded hello and displayed a thumbs-up for our longtime friendship and my fancy, but rumpled clothes. "Frank," I said, "if anyone comes asking for me, including a police sergeant, you haven't seen me."

I located clean scrubs and carefully hung my suit in the medical residents' office. It was too soon to take it to the cleaners, the food and coffee spots were not yet confluent.

The office was home to our undictated medical charts and miscellaneous stuff needed for correspondence, hospital-based or not. Scrunched-up letters to Sophie, not quite saying what I meant and never mailed, filled the corners of the room, missing the target wastebasket for the Dr. Howard versus Dr. Ted basketball endeavors, recently curtailed when I realized the students had posted my personal Sophie sentiments on the bulletin board. The cleaning people avoided the place, as the No Food And No Beverages, Clean Up Your Mess signs became a magnet for promoting the opposite.

Several sheets of carbon paper remained suffused with life, and I typed. And I typed some more, carefully describing the events of the past year: Betty's death, my two gangster friends, and the sudden turn of affairs involving my ex-buddy, Sergeant George Esposito, whom I now believed wanted me permanently gone.

"*Only read in case of my death or disappearance*," was a heck of a beginning. Agatha Christie would be proud, but there it was, heading my letter and prominently displayed in block letters on the front of the envelope. The ending of the epistle was also intriguing: "*This letter has no cross-outs, deletions or additions*." A nice touch to my discourse, I thought.

I walked down to the lobby, the hospital quietly awaiting the sunrise rush of chest pain and pre-op surgical business, and inserted change in the stamp machine that generously provided three four-cent stamps for a quarter. The usury was forgiven because of the choices. This morning it was the periwinkle-blue Arctic Explorations stamp, incongruously picturing both a submarine and a dog sled, or the taupe-brown Pony Express celebration. I chose the latter, the horse and rider going full-speed-ahead. It's a guy thing. I mailed one letter each to Stan Glicke, Howard, and Mrs. Gail. The latter recipient took some thought, but who better to serve justice than the fearless Mrs. Gail.

Telephoning Howard came next. He understood immediately and was ready to roll. I paged Sergeant Esposito, his reply quick, and asked him to meet me at the hospital cafeteria at seven a.m.

Monday morning, the cafeteria was busy, as hospital workers were early risers and the shift changed at this ungodly hour. And today, being the fourth Monday of the month, it was Luau Day. Starving after the long night, I joined the festivities and added a cup of pineapple bits and maraschino cherries to my Cheerios.

George, haggard and irritable looking, was not used to staying up all night. His hair combed too straight, thick and soft from the night's rain, the darkness billowing under his eyes featuring enough bags for a European vacation. What a contrast he was to the bright, ebullient me, shaved, showered, fed, and ready for battle.

Mrs. B brought the policeman coffee. It was self-service for me. "If you're going to arrest the doctor," she said, smiling angelically, "let me cuff him for you." And why not? Her favorite policeman was here, Hawaiian music flowed from the background speakers, and her bedraggled lei with white-and-rose colored plastic flower petals alternating with Monopoly dice jingled around her neck. Who needed grass skirts and poi when a handsome policeman attended your island party?

"Mrs. B, please, listen carefully," I interrupted her, touching her arm, speaking over the loudspeakers. "There's been a change in the dynamics between the sergeant and me. He's not the good guy anymore. He's not one of the righteous. There's no arrest warrant for me; he's a renegade. You'll need to take sides. It's me or him, and I need your help. If the bad sergeant pulls out his handcuffs or gun, please call hospital security, Jane, the hospital lawyer, and the police department. And keep an eye on us, would you please? I don't want any accidents messing up your beautiful cafeteria."

"Yes, Doctor, I'll do that," Mrs. B said after the briefest pause. Maybe it was asking her to telephone the police department about the sergeant that grabbed her attention.

"Mr. Policeman, the coffee is twenty-five cents, no refills, and we don't accept nothing larger than a five-dollar bill," and she held out her hand for payment.

"Thank you, Mrs. B," I said.

Howard sitting quietly several tables away, acknowledged the goings-on with a nod.

"George, I just mailed out the 'open only if something happens to me,' letters. Unfortunately, I ran out of carbon paper, so you won't receive a copy, but let me bring you into the loop." I worked at my little speech, shifting around in my armless chair, the awkwardness between ex-friends straining at both of us. "I assume you're not wearing a wire—no don't undress here, Mrs. B might become orgasmic. I don't think you're working for people who employ stoolies, and just for safety's sake, mine mainly, Howard, my buddy, is keeping track of our negotiations."

George was sitting upright and stiff as if posing for a daguerreotype portrait by Mathew Brady, dour, fatigued with steely dark eyes fixed on mine, a Union soldier perhaps, contemplating a bleak future while remembering his fallen comrades.

"There were only two things that could have gone wrong when I shot Tim. One is those unavoidable events that occur without warning or reason. Someone walks in when you're pulling the trigger, someone recognizes you on the street, a patient, a relative, a friend—or maybe you show up in someone's picture-taking moment, those random happenings that spoil good intentions. You're a cop; you know about those things."

The sergeant, sitting motionless, remained mute.

"The other is you, George. You're one of the few who knew my motive and the only one with the resources to decipher my gun purchases.

"Let me tell you about that.

"The gun that killed Tim was wrapped in plastic wrap, you know, the kind that fits snug around the handle like magic. You have to pry it loose with a chisel. Because of that stuff, the pistol doesn't have my fingerprints on it. That gun can be found. I know exactly where it's at. And so do the people I've sent the letters to including Stan Glicke."

The turn of events wasn't settling pleasantly with the tired detective, who was fidgeting around in his chair, his tongue absentmindedly working over his right upper molars. Not being able to floss at night takes its toll.

"Exciting, right, the gun that killed mob boss Tim Schmidt is found intact. It'll finally solve a mob murder, because smack-dab on the handle, underneath the wrap, are perfect fingerprints. The kind of prints—and I'm speaking literally—are ones you can die for. The 'you' is you of course. Granted, they were lifted from a coffee cup with Scotch tape and then planted on the handle, but hey, that's a secret just between the two of us.

"What's happening in this world," people will exclaim. Sergeant George Esposito's fingerprints on the murder weapon! I know he was going after Tim Schmidt, but murdering him?

"I'm aghast, aren't you also, Mr. Detective?"

In spite of my damning monologue—the sergeant's mood seemed to be recovering. Specks of a smile were blossoming, more in his eyes than around his mouth.

"I thought about placing Mr. Baseball's prints on the gun. Now, wouldn't that be wonderful and also solve a lot of murders? But he was too much fun for me to set up like that. Who would I go to baseball games with? His mixture of violence and humor make me smile," I said, thinking that Mr. Baseball actually reminded me of myself.

"George it's you I worry about. Stan told me you were trouble. You told the thugs to go after me and when that failed, there you were waiting in my apartment to do me harm. Do you have an alibi on the night that Tim was killed?" I asked him with renewed confidence, crossing my legs and sitting back in my chair. "If you don't, you've got a real problem. I'm not willing to be a fall guy for a piece of shit like Tim, and unless you want to take the rap, I'd suggest you keep away from me. Find someone else to bother, or knock off, and get out of my life. And forget about that Tomczak thing—I'll tell the authorities you were setting me up."

Pleased with my dissertation, I stopped, wiggled my torso for comfort, moistened my throat with coffee, and let George carry the ball.

"Doc," George was becoming more alert, stretching the muscles of his back, his eyes meeting mine again, speaking slowly and carefully—"listen to me for a few minutes.

"Tim Schmidt was one of *our* guys, working for us undercover. A mole! An important mole! Why in the hell do you think you received so much attention for your crazy notion about Betty's death, when there were hundreds of real murders needing to be solved every year in our city?"

Time stopped for me, but not for George. It was his turn and maybe he was sailing the prizewinning sloop.

"And me Doc, believe it or not, I'm okay. I'm infiltrating them—the mob.

"Then you come along out of nowhere and kill our number-one stoolie, and probably for no good reason. Tim, as mean as he was, wouldn't have killed his wife. These guys may be crazy, but wife-killing is not part of their temperament. Doc, let me tell you something I learned in the police academy. It's scientific. You'll understand what I'm saying, what with all of your schooling and book smarts. Attachment theory! It's called attachment theory. The perps use it all the time! They find an alibi they like, and they repeat it to themselves so many times that it becomes the truth to them.

"You believed Tim killed his wife, no matter what anyone said to you, including the lupus expert from the university, and your own pathologist. Even after the autopsy findings, you still never would let go.

"I'm told by the evil guys to settle the score for Tim's death. An eye for an eye.

No deed goes unpunished. The police brass said to go-ahead. It's for the general good. It'll cement my standing with the gangsters.

"Sorry to inform you, but even a doctor is a pawn in our wars.

"But you're not just a doctor. You're a vigilante—a murderer. Once you killed Tim, you moved to a different part of the city. The dark side. You became fair game for a lot of bad things."

The pause lingered longer than I would have thought possible. Was the sergeant telling the truth?

"Hopefully, I have enough clout to call off my assignment to take you out," George finally said. "I would like that. And by the way, Doc, fingerprints really can't be transferred. Tape absorbs the oil and grime that make up the print, and those prints won't stick on the ridged metal of a handgun.

"Your planning was almost perfect. But now you've given me a chance to work this out with my bosses without more violence. The possibility of the murder weapon with my accidental fingerprints on it—smart! I'll play it as a legitimate setup, and we'll solve Tim's murder another way without involving my favorite doc.

"Ted, my friend, you're in the wrong profession. Jesus, you're thinking like a pro, a mechanic, and you're a goddamn doc.

"The summer pool parties and beer and hotdogs at my place—you're always invited. My wife's pretty little sister, an Elizabeth Taylor twin, likes her men smart and tough—ignore her divorces, the men were too rough. The two of you will meld as one—you'll see. I'll set it up.

"It's almost been a pleasure," the sergeant finished. "Oh, and it might be best to try to retrieve your letters." The tiredness was breaking through again. A frozen smile appeared, the kind seen on the receptionists at a Motel 6.

With that the sergeant pried himself up and left. Not waiting to hear the truth. Tim had killed Betty. I was sure of it.

I also departed, nodding at Mrs. B and offering her one of my best smiles. I was the happy, young, cooperative man on the go she'd now respect and hopefully accept his on-call coupons without a fuss. Such a contrast he was to the mean-looking and tired policeman who had just left. Howard joined me. I gave him the all-okay smile, and said nothing about the possibility that I might have killed an innocent man.

# THIRTEEN

*A Little Madness in the Spring*
*Is wholesome even for the King.*

*~Emily Dickinson*

The story was hidden in the local news. It should have been in the sports section. Nikolai V was found dead in the hospital jail. He had been recovering from his gunshot wounds. The bullet crushed his ribs, but was deflected away from the lung and heart. The good fortune was short-lived. The cause of death was not mentioned.

"Nikolai V, an immigrant from Russia with ties to the Chicago mob, previously made headline news because of his major league baseball aspirations that were cut short when he attacked his manager with his favorite bat. He was the chief suspect in the murder of Tim Schmidt, a mobster and recent victim…"

The latter was news to me, but I guess in the perverted world of organized crime, with cops in pursuit, he was as good a patsy as any other. Rest in peace, Nikolai V, and may your eternity include a batter's cage.

❖ ❖ ❖

The end-of-the-year, promotion, going-away, release-your-pent-up angst party, was the highlight of our year.

For the IntMed 3s, it was a time for major transitions. Private practice opportunities, specialized training, marriages, divorces, births, moving—decisions best left to the young.

Plus, there were other important things: Howard and I had to organize the entertainment for the party. Nothing gentle either, like our sudden and inexplicable soft spot for Estelle and Fineglass.

Amy, my date, understood upfront that she wouldn't be sitting at the chief's table. It was back to pedestrian days. Graceful on her feet, Amy owned a good voice because after performing our Mr. Ray Show—and believe me, it was difficult to get a puppet to play the accordion. We sang a medley of stupid songs, pipe smoked through our nose, name-called, judged a castanet-playing marathon, and a one-legged tap-dancing contest—the works.

For me, it was time to say goodbye to my criminal past. George, my new nemesis couldn't be trusted, although the funny thing was, I still liked him. I liked Mr. Baseball also—*Spoczywaj w spokoju*, rest in peace, Nikolai V. More to the point, they both could have been my Friday night poker and Saturday night cruising buddies.

Mother and Father always wished me sweet sleep at bedtime. Not sweet dreams. I thought it was their foreign-born jumbled notion. Dreams were sometimes sweet and sometimes not, they told me after the goodnight kisses. But, sleep, they said, always left you happy. They were right. It was the twilight border between sleep and awakening with the lingering headaches that were the problem, because right and wrong seemed to merge in that place. But maybe that too will pass and maybe I'll settle down and pay attention to advice and discipline and let injustices slip by, although, that said, I probably won't.

The End

# *Acknowledgements*

My gratitude to…
Fred Shafer and Julie West Johnson—
my writing instructors; and my many supportive and skilled compadres,
especially the steadfast writers and critics from the
Wilmette Library Writing Group—my heartfelt thanks.

Made in the USA
Monee, IL
20 November 2025

35675049R00163